Fight Like a Mother

How to Be a Mom With a Chronic Illness

By
Joslyne C. Decker

For My Mom,
My hero.

CONTENTS

WITH GRATITUDE

Thank you to all those who encouraged me to write this book, including: Tyffany, Amy Lyles Wilson, Lisa McKay, Alicia, Ron R. and Damaris. Uncle Thomas, thanks for your editing eye. Chip and Holly, thank you for making me feel like a real writer. And thanks again to Lisa for hooking me up. Special love for my chronically ~~ill~~ awesome readers: Aunt Janet, Alicia, and Kate. Thanks to everyone who helped me keep going over the years, especially: Tyffany (you're in here twice – you're a STAR!), Niki, Kate M., Kate C., Carrie, Courtney, Susan, Nancy, and the TN playgroup. Super thanks to my Mom and Dad who are the best parents in the whole universe. Demetri and Zoey, thank you for Every. Single. Thing. You are my favorites. xo.

INTRODUCTION:
SO, YOU HAVE A LIFE CHANGING CHRONIC ILLNESS
(sympathetic head tilt)

I spend a fair amount of time wishing I was a super hero. I guess flying and invisibility would be nice super powers to have, but I wish for something else. Super strength to lift more than 10 pounds on a consistent basis! Super speed to walk two blocks without pain! Super stamina to stay awake past 8:30 p.m.! Also, I have a thing for capes. I imagine wearing a cape is like wearing a blanket – I could nap anywhere!

I'm tired of the limits of my chronic illnesses – fibromyalgia and depression. I'm tired of wishing I was a super hero. So I've decided to just *be* one. In fact, I'm building an army of super heroes. And you're totally invited. We won't have the usual super powers (yawn): telekinesis, flight, or the freakish ability to wield one of the basic elements (although if I could, I would totally pick water). Instead, we will have more, um, *specialized* super powers.

I know someone with IBS who can hold in her poo until she finds a bathroom. The willpower and muscle strength this takes is astounding. She also happens to have the super powers of lifting heavy things and accidentally making up good t-shirt slogans. I know someone with Lupus who makes these seriously amazing Christmas ornaments . . . with her bare hands. I have another friend who suffers from depression, knows all the words to "American Pie", and has run two half marathons. Someone else I know with fibromyalgia is able to show gratitude for the small and big things in life Every. Single. Day. Another friend with SOD type II not only has the sharpest wit EVER, but the ability to make perfect flowers out of frosting. Plus, she says she can do kegels like a ninja. Despite my chronic illnesses, I am really good at lip-synching to '80's pop ballads. Also, I can get the damn horse back riding boots on the knock-off "American Girl" dolls from Target. In case you've never done it, I assure you it's TOTALLY a super power.

So, if you put us all together you have a poo-holding, heavy-lifting and t-shirt-slogan-making, craft-creating, half marathon running, gratitude-giving, wit-wielding-and-edible-flower-making, '80's-lip-synching, kegel-ninja-ing FORCE. Even The Hulk couldn't take us.

Come and join our army of Super Heroes. Because even though you have a chronic illness, you also have a super powers. WE NEED YOU!

Like I said, I have depression and fibromyalgia. In case you don't know, fibromyalgia is a chronic illness "characterized by widespread musculoskeletal pain accompanied by fatigue, sleep, memory and mood issues."[1] Fibromyalgia, like many other chronic illnesses, can also be isolating, frustrating, and painful. But, then again, I get to take lots of naps and I will never have to help anyone move ever again.

Besides being one of the 133 million Americans with a chronic illness[2], I'm also mom to 5-year-old Zoey. Zoey is often described as "spirited" and "independent." I am told I will appreciate these qualities even more when she is older. I like to describe Zoey as "42 pounds of awesome."

I was diagnosed with fibromyalgia before I was a mom. First, in 2006, then I was re-diagnosed in 2008 by a fibromyalgia expert, and re-re-diagnosed in 2012 by another expert. Although I experienced some depression in college, my diagnosis of major depressive disorder coincided with my diagnosis of fibromyalgia. Being told you will live a life of pain and fatigue, in a pain-med induced haze tends to bring a

---

[1] Mayo Clinic Staff. "Definition." *Diseases and Conditions: Fibromyalgia.* Accessed January 22, 2011. http://www.mayoclinic.org/diseases-
conditions/fibromyalgia/basics/definition/CON-20019243
[2] "About Chronic Diseases." *nationalhealthcouncil.org.* Last modified April 11, 3013.
http://www.nationalhealthcouncil.org/NHC_Files/Pdf_Files/AboutChronicDisease.pdf

person down. Thankfully the doctor who told me that was a little bit dumb, or to put it more generously, he was wrong.

I am grateful for my body — it is young and strong in many ways. My body has been good to me. It's played in hundreds of soccer games. It's run a half marathon; it's hiked, swum, and biked. It's even turned into the body of a mom — a body that sings and wipes and soothes and cleans and feeds and hugs and does a million other things for someone else. But often my body is tired. Sore. I feel bent and broken in ways other people don't.

I should not have to eat small bites of oatmeal in the morning because a regular size spoonful is too heavy. I should not have to listen to Zoey cry because I can't pick her up. I should not have to ask my dad to accompany me to the grocery store so he can lift the items off the shelf for me — graham crackers, apple juice, marinara sauce. The pain and fatigue is always there – sometimes a lightweight and gauzy sweater, sometimes chainmail. Just like the weather, it's always changing, moving from one thing to the next.

Mostly I am lucky. I choose not to live my life in a pain-med induced haze. I run. I let Zoey crawl into my lap and I kiss her cheek. I lift a fragrant, ripe cantaloupe. I have people who love me. People who do the motions of life for me when I can't. People who forgive my anger and meanness about being sick — whether it's directed towards them or towards myself. Mostly I am okay. Mostly I am well enough. But when I'm not — oh, how it hurts! Not just my body, also my heart.

I've read my fair share of books and articles about fibromyalgia and found most of them to be soul-sucking. I felt worse after reading them. True, there was that one I threw in the fireplace, which made it slightly harder to finish. It might have rallied to become witty and uplifting in the last few chapters, but probably not.

Often books on chronic illness are written by "experts," or at least someone who works at a hospital or something. These writers have a whole lot of concern for us and our "life-changing chronic illness." They write softly because, apparently, we are upset easily. They pat our hands, tilt their heads, and look out at us from their dust jacket covers with wide, moist Bambi eyes assuring us that they get it. They understand. They urge us to creep through life with care, planning, and extra blankets. These authors leave out practical advice, like how to get someone to lift something for us and how to use memory loss to our advantage. Plus, most authors assume we don't have kids. These books would drive me to drink if drinking was something my fibromyalgia allowed. Sadly, I have to drown my sorrows in de-caffeinated tea.

So much of the advice out there isn't realistic for moms. At least for moms without nannies, maids, and chauffeurs. These other books may have some good advice. I just don't appreciate the narrowness of the advice and how it's often given. You know, the condescending voice advising us to get ten hours of uninterrupted sleep every night and to put on make-up every day so we feel "pretty." Ugh. I think these "experts" don't get it, but rather have researched it, read about it, and talked to people with it. *Knowing about it* and *getting it* are two completely different things.

So, you were daring and bought a book not written by a medical professional, or researcher. High-five! But gently, please (because of the whole fibromyalgia thing). Over the years I've figured out what helps me by trial and error, by finding a few good medical professionals, and by talking to others with chronic illness about their experiences. This book offers some advice. And some cautionary tales. But it will also make you laugh. Or snort. Mostly you will be laughing at me. No, no, not with me. *At me.* You can mock my funny failures! You can learn from my mistakes! If you're a mom with a chronic illness, you can take heart in knowing that there are moms out there who have been where you are — newly diagnosed, unceremoniously dumped out of the doctor's office (don't you think we should at least be given a tiara or something?) and wondering, "Chronicwhatnow?" You don't have to go into uncharted territory alone. You definitely don't have to proceed with solemnity and stoicism.

Take a breath.

Grab some chocolate.

Keep going.

1

CHRONIC-SCHMONIC

When I am sad, I stop being sad and be awesome instead.
-Barney Stinson (Neil Patrick Harris),
How I Met Your Mother

Not to brag or anything, but when I was first diagnosed with fibromyalgia I was very brave. I was the epitome of grace and inspiration. I walked around with really good hair and a nice butt — the kind that looks good in yoga pants. When I slowly sashayed by, people would whisper, "Look at her! She has a life-changing chronic illness *and* a shapely derriere! What a vision!" And ever since then I have been inspiring the masses with my good hair, curvaceous booty, and amazing attitude.

Not so much.

I have flat hair and a flat ass. A back-with-a-crack. A no-butt. Also, I was like most other people in the world and went through the messy stages of grief[3] when diagnosed with a chronic illness. But to ease ourselves in, let's go through the steps as if we suddenly had no access to chocolate.

- **Denial.** "I'm sure there's chocolate somewhere!"
- **Anger.** "I'm pissed there's no chocolate!"
- **Bargaining.** "I'll never swear again if I find some chocolate!"

---

[3] Kubler-Ross, Elisabeth. "On Death and Dying." (New York: Scribner, 1969).

- **Depression.** "There's no chocolate and I'm a horrible person."
- **Acceptance.** "There's no chocolate and I can deal with it. Probably."

Yup, these stages aren't just for losing a loved one. They also work for any major life loss — like being diagnosed with a chronic illness. Not everyone goes through the steps the same way — some people skip steps, and there's no set sequence. "The stages are responses to feelings that can last for minutes or hours as we flip in and out of one and then another."[4]

I did depression at least twice. I skipped bargaining. Probably because I spent such a long time in the anger and depression stages. Or because I'm so advanced.

Denial

"Denial helps us to pace our feelings of grief. There is a grace in denial. It is nature's way of letting in only as much as we can handle." [5]

Welcome to my first stage of grief when faced with a chronic illness. Can I serve you a hot, steaming bowl of denial? Lots and lots of denial. Here's how the "conversation" about fibromyalgia went with my doctor the first time I was diagnosed. I use the word "conversation" loosely as I said nothing, and sat there with tears and snot streaming down my face, too tired to reach for a tissue.

What the doctor actually said (as confirmed by my husband, Demetri, who was present):

"So, it appears you have fibromyalgia. Fibromyalgia is a condition characterized by pain all over your body, tender points, fatigue, and poor sleep. It can be triggered by stress or a physical injury. You should probably quit your highly stressful job. Do you want a bunch of pain meds?"

---

[4] "The Five Stages of Grief The responses to Grief that Many People Have." *Grief.com*. Retrieved June 28, 2013. http://grief.com/the-five-stages-of-grief/
[5] ibid

What I heard:

"You are not really sick. You are a wimp. You are, in fact, the biggest wimp I have ever seen in 28 years of practicing medicine. Also, you are lazy. You just need to apply yourself and work hard. It is my conclusion, and the conclusion of everyone in this office, that you are a bad person. You have a flat ass and bad hair. Do you want a bunch of pain meds?"

In short, I viewed my chronic illness as a personality "issue" instead of a medical condition. I viewed it as something I could change. I felt like the secret I held for so long was out — my family and friends now all knew, knew *for sure*, that I was lazy, weak, and unreliable. I didn't try hard enough. I was a quitter.

I thought about all the things I had done in life that were maybe not so good: I told my husband he looked okay in a mock turtleneck; I got a C in ceramics class in college; when I was six, I sold lemonade made out of gutter water to neighborhood kids and then my mom had to go door to door to make sure none of the kids were poisoned. Clearly, I could be better in so many ways — a better person, a better friend, a better daughter, a better wife. I just needed to suck it up and be like everyone else: energetic, strong, capable.

So I tried becoming a better person. A nicer person. A well person. Instead, I became depressed.

Depression

"If grief is a process of healing, then depression is one of the many necessary steps along the way." [6]

Somehow on my quest to be a better person, I couldn't manage to get out of bed very often. Or leave the house. Not that one can't do good in the world as a bedridden recluse with poor personal hygiene, but those characteristics seem to hinder rather than help. So I stayed in bed, cried, and thought about how my laziness was a drain on my friends and family. I

---

[6] ibid

3

thought about Demetri and how he married me just two months before. He thought he married a vibrant, hot chick who could lift more than 15 pounds and could use a can opener. Now, in a matter of weeks, he was hitched to a sniveling weakling with a life-changing chronic illness. And I still had a flat ass.

Demetri, my kind husband who, by the way, has a very nice ass, just smiled and laughed when I asked if he was going to leave me because of either (a) my lack of a butt, (b) my laziness, (c) the fact that I hadn't showered in four days.

I gradually stopped crying so much. I showered more. I left the house sometimes. All while continuing to think that my problem was I was a bad person. I did two stages at once: denial and depression. I am a fantastic multi-tasker. Booya!

Occasionally I felt a tiny whisper of a thought, "Maybe, just maybe, I have an illness. Maybe fibromyalgia is real." I brushed away the thought. I brushed it away because if I was a bad person I could actually change that. But if I had a chronic illness, well, that might be something I couldn't change.

Then I got mad.

Anger

"Anger is a necessary stage of the healing process. Be willing to feel your anger, even though it may seem endless. The more you truly feel it, the more it will begin to dissipate and the more you will heal." [7]

Welcome to the anger stage. RAWR! Instead of being all noble and strong, I became like a two-year-old who just had her lollipop taken away. I felt like a big, angry baby with no frustration tolerance, very few brains, and absolutely no ability to think beyond myself. Never mind people who don't have clean water. Or homes. I had been struck down and I didn't deserve it! It wasn't fair.

So I took my anger out on everything and everyone,

---

[7] ibid

4

especially those people/things living in the same house as me. Which meant Demetri. The poor guy took a metaphorical beating. Once, there was even an attempted real beating.

Demetri and I were standing in the living room, face-to-face, arguing about, you know, something, when suddenly my anger surged to new levels. All the unfairness, pain, and despair funneled down to this moment.

I launched myself across the living room directly at my husband, yelling, "Hiiiiiii-YAAAAAAA!" I aimed a mid-air karate kick at Demetri's nether regions . . . which sadly/luckily (depending on who you ask) fell short. My wild karate kick leap only got me about two feet across the room instead of the five feet I needed to go to reach my target. Damn the fatigue!

I let out a new war cry, "Wrestle me weakling!" I ran, head down and arms flailing, at Demetri.

He looked a bit panicked, backed up to the wall, and said, "Honeeeeey! Nooooo!"

As I pulled him to the ground, he yelled, "I don't want to hurt you!"

"Ha," I sputtered in his face. "HA!"

Before I could blink, he pinned my arms to my sides, immobilized my legs with some sort of ninja flip-scissor-kick move, and sat on top of me.

"I don't want to wrestle you," he said calmly.

"That's. Because." I grunted as I attempted to struggle free, "I'm. Beating. You."

You might think I would act more like an adult, stop struggling, and get up off the floor. You would be wrong. I struggled until I was worn out. Until I was exhausted and spent. It was a long seven seconds.

Demetri held my arms and sat on me in the kindest possible way until I gave up. I felt charred — burnt up and empty. So full of nothing that I could blow away, I could be pinched into meaningless dust. Demetri slid off me and tried to cup my face gently in his hands. I couldn't bear to look at him — his soft eyes, the creases around his mouth when he smiled, his familiarity. I rolled over, buried my face in the

5

carpet, and cried. I couldn't hold it in; I couldn't hold myself together. I cried because I was so tired. I cried out of humiliation. I cried because I didn't know how to have fibromyalgia *and* be myself. "F*** you fibromyalgia," I thought.

I wish I could write here about how I immediately moved on to the acceptance stage of the grieving process, about how my acceptance changed my illness and my life. But that's not what happened. Instead, I landed smack in the middle of depression. Again.

Welcome back to even worse fashion sense than usual, carbs, and bad romantic comedies meant for a much younger age group. I thought it was a great idea to wear the same charcoal gray sweat pants, eat a lot of toast, and watch *13 Going on 30* and *The Princess Diaries*. Every day. Also, I didn't really leave the house. I cried a lot. I went to bed at seven p.m.

Acceptance

"Acceptance is often confused with the notion of being "all right" or "OK" with what has happened. This is not the case. . . Finding acceptance may be just having more good days than bad ones . . . ." [8]

Eventually, there is a stage called acceptance. It's not a constant state of being. It's more like flashes of accepting moments: moments of progress, moments of ease, moments of feeling like whatever we are is enough.

Several years ago, when I went to see yet another fibromyalgia specialist, I got schooled in my big picture version of acceptance. I learned that my "acceptance" was rather non-existent. I was afraid (and ashamed) that the specialist would tell me I didn't have fibromyalgia, that I was just lazy and weak. I was afraid he would confirm that the whole chronic illness thing was my fault. However, the specialist confirmed the diagnosis of fibromyalgia and added chronic fatigue and severe iron deficiency.

---

[8] ibid

When I went to see the doctor I feared he would tell me, "Well, golly, no. No, you don't have fibromyalgia. You're just a big wimp. Now go out and be better!" When he didn't tell me that, I realized *not* having fibromyalgia was a fear . . . and a hope. A hope that maybe I was okay, normal, fine. I'm not *not* those things. But I'm not fully those things either. I'm in-between.

At first, I was angry at being banished to The In-Between. I was angry at being sent there forever. I was bitter and scared and falling apart. But only a little. I realized the In-Between is my version of acceptance.

Most of the time The In-Between is not a terrible place to be. It can be a little grey and a little lonely. But I'm making myself a room here. With yellow curtains and a braided rug. A tea pot with fading roses painted on the side. Books. A rocking chair. A green and heather knitted blanket. I am learning to be comfortable here. I am learning to live in this new space of being unwell.

Truth be told, I fought against this idea of learning to be unwell for a long time. I shoved it aside with scorn and anger declaring, "What the (insert swear word of choice)!!! I don't want to learn to be sick! *I* want to learn to be *well*!"

Now I think I have to do both. I need to learn how to catch the wave of wellness when I can. And I need to learn how to batten down the hatches and be . . . unwell. I need to learn to be unwell the best that I can, because all this struggling against my illnesses, all this turning against myself, is killing me. I don't know for sure, but I suspect that learning to be unwell is a skill. I suspect that learning to be unwell while still participating in my life with love, patience, and meaning is the best way to fight. I also suspect it takes a lot of practice.

My acceptance is a work in progress. I bask in it when it's there and, when it's gone, I trust I can gently pull it back to me.

Bargaining

"We become lost in a maze of "If only…" or "What if…" statements. We want life returned to what it was… Guilt is often bargaining's companion."[9]

I wrote earlier that I skipped the bargaining stage. Well, that was a total lie. I must have been in denial. I often think about the things I wish I could do. I dream about what my life, relationships, and career would be like if only I didn't have fibromyalgia and depression. And it's just now, after seven years of this wishful thinking, that I'm learning to let it go. I am where I am. Right now I'm trying to stay in the moment – whether it's painful or joyful – because it will eventually change into something else. And, really, I am also here because I have no choice. I have fibromyalgia.

So, what about you? Maybe you're thinking, "Well, crap. I thought all I had to do was deal with my chronic illness, and now I have to deal with all these stages as well?" If you're thinking something with more swear words, it probably means you're already at the anger stage. Congratulations! If you're thinking, "Hey, I just got diagnosed and it's aaallllll good." You are either (a) in the acceptance stage — try not to brag too much, or (b) in denial. Wherever you are right now, know that tomorrow, or in ten minutes, you may be somewhere different. That's okay. It just means you're doing it right — you're being human. Wherever you are, here are some tips to get you through.

---

[9] ibid

Chronically Awesome[10] Tips:
Adjusting to a Chronic Illness Diagnosis

- **Don't wrestle anyone.** Enough said.

- **You can only be where you are.** Be loosely aware of the previous stages and let your body and mind do what they need to do. You can encourage yourself along:
  - not good: "I'm stupid, which is why I'm stuck in the depression phase."
  - good: "One day I will feel more accepting of my illness than I do now. That day is not today, and that's okay."

- **Don't go it alone.** Ask for help. Make sure you get it. Trust me, these stages are better and shorter if you let someone walk with you, even just part of the way.

- **Have a good primary care doctor and a good therapist.** Use them.

- **Don't initiate any major life changes.** Adjusting to your chronic illness and figuring out how to feel your best is enough. For example, don't decide to embark on a new career or take up roller derby just after being diagnosed.

- **Have good snacks.** This is just good general life advice.

---

[10] "Chronically Awesome" is a servicemark and copywrite of The Chronically Awesome Foundation (http://chronicallyawesome.org/) and is used with permission.

NOW WHAT??

The first step is always the hardest,
but it's the only way to reach the second step.
- Susan Gale

The first time I was diagnosed with fibromyalgia, my doctor told me to quit my job and gave me three different prescriptions for pain medication. That was it. He didn't even give me a badly photocopied sheet with sleep advice and stretching tips. It was a total rip-off. He also didn't offer me a goodbye tissue as I walked out the door crying.

Demetri drove me home, his hand on my knee. At that moment, his hand was the only thing keeping me there – the only thing keeping me from shriveling up into nothing and being blown away. I focused so hard on his hand — the weight, the strength, the promise that he was with me, and that I was real. When we got home I curled up on the couch and cried. All I could think was, "Now what?"

For the next few weeks I couldn't do anything. I was too fatigued and too overwhelmed. It took all the energy I had to move from room to room and occasionally put chocolate in my mouth. Then two things happened: my mom came to stay with me for a few days, and I went for a walk with my best friend of 30 years. When my mom came, she cooked for me and she sat with me when I didn't even have the energy to talk. She made me feel safe. My beautiful, wonderful mother gave me the first glimmer of hope that things might be okay.

About a week after being diagnosed, right around the time I quit my job and we realized we were going to have to move to a place with cheaper rent, my friend Tyffany came over and took me for a walk. She picked me up, drove me to the arboretum, and told me to get the hell out of the car. My goal was to walk a mile, something that had previous been no big deal. We walked — slowly and carefully. I still felt so tired and fragile. Tyffany is a competitive person. She's been known to topple over a Scrabble board when losing, and she likes to do things fast, crazy, and adventurous. I have never been able to keep up with her on a bike or on foot. I usually just wave to her as she is climbing rocks and doing pop-a-wheelies. But on this particular day she walked with me, exactly at my pace. I'm sure it practically killed her. We walked for 25 minutes and still hadn't finished the mile; we took a shortcut back to the car. What I remember from that day is the brightness of the flowers in full spring bloom, the blue of the sky, and the feeling of having someone walk beside me, our elbows occasionally bumping and our feet in exact rhythm.

Now what?

Now it's your turn to join the club of Chronic Super Heroes. Condolences and welcome! You've been diagnosed with a chronic illness. You're wondering, "Now what?" Well, right now you are going to give yourself a few days to grieve, to shake your fist at the sky, and to sleep. You are going to mobilize your support systems. Then you are going to get up and fight.

Yes, you *are* going to get up and fight. I can feel it. You may be fighting to get well. You may be fighting for the energy to play Pretty Princess Glitter Fairies with your child. You may be fighting to keep a sense of yourself throughout your illness. You may be fighting to get through the afternoon. No matter what it is, know that you are worth fighting for. And know that you need some help.

Chronically Awesome Tips:
How to Get *Helpful* Help

• **Decide WHAT you need.**
Ask for specific help. If you don't, you won't get what
you need. In fact, you might get some things you really
don't want, like unsolicited advice. People want to help
but they often don't know *how* to help. Here are some
ideas on what you may need help with and how to ask:

Meals	"We could really use a dinner on Wednesday night."
Groceries	"If you're going to the store, would you please grab me some string cheese and chocolate?"
Rides to appointments	"Would you please drop me off at the doctor's on your way to the store?"
School pick up or drop off	"I'd really appreciate it if Sylvia could catch a ride to school with you."
Child care	"If you could take little Julian for two hours that would be so helpful."
Outings for your kids	"Hey, can little Lily come with you to the park?"
A walking buddy	"Can you come over and take me for a 15 minute walk? I know I won't do it alone."
Yard work	"If you could spend 30 minutes mowing our front yard that would be incredible!"
Cleaning	"You would be my hero if you vacuumed my living room!"
A shopping buddy	"Can you drive me to Target and then help me lift things into the cart?"
Company	"I would love to have someone just come over and hang out for 30 minutes."

- **Appoint a Magical Manager.** Under no circumstances are you to arrange and schedule all this help yourself. Ask a trusted friend to coordinate the help for you. Make sure this friend can say no: "No, Thursday afternoon is not a good time to visit." "No, she doesn't want to try kale brownies." Also ask this friend to keep track of who does what so you can thank everyone later. Having a Magical Manager is really important. Give her a tiara and the title of Magical Manager. Tell her what you need and when, then direct people to email her instead of you. If you do not do this, you will spend all your time answering emails and scheduling stuff and it will make you want to claw your eyes out. This is not helpful. Save your energy and let someone else manage it.

- **Use a free online signup to organize helpers.** Obviously, your Magical Manager should do this. These sites let your Magical Manager set up specific categories of need (including times and dates) and then allow people to sign up for what they can help with. The sites also allow easy communication between organizers and helpers (it sends automatic reminders etc.) — a huge time saver for your Magical Manager. Some sites I like include: signupgenius.com, carecalendar.org, www.mealtrain.com.

- **Use social media (Facebook, Twitter, etc.) to ASK for help.** Yeah, you actually have to ask. People post on Facebook stuff like, "The sun is out!" and "My dog pooped on the floor ☹," so it's okay to post that you need a bit of help. If you are not comfortable announcing your specific illness, just say you are feeling unwell and need some support. If social media is too public for you, use email. Or better yet, have your Magical Manager send out an email on your behalf. Social media can surprise you, though. People generally want to help if they can, so it's the best way to get the most help from the greatest number of people. You don't want to constantly tax the same small group of friends. A sample post: "Hey Fabulous Friends, Having a bit of a rough time right now. In need of meals, school pick-up, and groceries. I'll pay you back in chocolate and love. Please contact Tyffany Smith at tyff@email.com."

- **Do not allow people to just "pop" by.** Ask them to give a specific time or provide them with a specific time window. For example, "Between 3:00 and 3:30." Otherwise you can't rest and plan your day because you never know when someone will show up. Asking people to drop stuff on the doorstep is also a good idea. That way you don't feel like you have to entertain and they don't feel like they have to stay.

- **It's okay not to visit with everyone.** It is perfectly fine to give your magical manager a list of people you don't really want to see. When I'm at my worst, there are very few people that I am comfortable spending time with. Anyone else just causes me stress and anxiety.

- **Provide a list of food allergies, food likes and dislikes.** Give this list to your Magical Manager. It won't be helpful if someone brings over enchiladas and your kid makes gagging noises when asked to eat something smothered in sauce.

- **Give people an out.** Especially when asking for help on an individual basis. For example, send an email and begin with: "I am writing to ask you a favor. If you aren't able to do it, I totally understand. (Then add some kind of compliment here like, "I've so appreciated all your help in the past.")

How the heck do I feel better?

A not-so-awesome fact: There is no universal way to feel better. What works for me may cause crushing pain or fatigue for you. (Yet another reason to shake our fists at the sky.) So, what we have to do when first diagnosed is try things, one at a time, until we find what works for us.

This is a pain in the ass. It's slow. It's frustrating. And, I'll be honest, not everything we try will help. Some of our attempts will be humiliating (see section on swimming). But here's the clincher: It's worth it. It's worth it to feel better than we do when first diagnosed, to feel a bit more in control, and to feel like we can work with our bodies instead of in spite of them.

Don't worry. I've totally got your back. Below is a list of things that may help in controlling symptoms like pain, fatigue, and poor sleep. Chronic illness can also cause depression, anxiety, memory loss, and stress. Yup, chronic illnesses can cause . . . wait for it . . . chronic illness. Whoever set that up clearly should be fired. I am not including specific medications, supplements, or diets on this list; it's best to work with a medical doctor or naturopath in those arenas.

So. The list. Put a check mark next to an item if you are even kinda-maybe-sorta interested in exploring it as a way of managing your health. Be sure and check at least one form of exercise because if you don't do it now, your doctor will make you do it sooner or later. There will be more on exercising later in the book. Spoiler alert! I fall off a bike and a balance ball.

Okay. Pretend I am holding your hand while you look over the list — your non check-marking hand. Pretend I am whispering in your ear in a reassuring way. Pretend I have really good cinnamon-y breath: "It's okay. You can do this."

Things that may help as part of a regular routine:	Things that may help occasionally	Things to avoid:
Walking	Whining	Stress
Jogging	Sniveling	Caffeine
Swimming	Cursing	Alcohol
Biking	Online shopping	Smoking
TheraBands	Chocolate	Negative Self Talk
Exercise Ball	Staying in bed	Being a recluse
Yoga	Heating pads	
Pilates	Staring at a wall	
Tai Chi	Mindless TV	
Strength training	Good movies	
Acupressure or acupuncture	Good books	
Dietary changes (speak with your doctor)	Online support group	
Therapeutic massage		
Physical therapy		
Talk therapy		
Meditation		
Chiropractic work		
Naps		
Transcranial Magnetic Stimulation		
Medication		

It's okay to be overwhelmed. It's okay to be scared. But don't let the fear keep you from trying things. At least one thing on this list will help you. Really, it will. Pick one thing, just one. Try it. If it causes major pain, stop.

For example, if it's exercise, start slow. Walk for a few minutes a minutes a day three times a week for a few weeks. Gradually increase your time. Then reevaluate. When you find something that helps, you'll know it. Jump gently for joy! Celebrate with cake! Or a nap! But whatever you do, make that thing — the thing that helps — part of your regular routine.

3

TALKING ABOUT IT

*When you don't talk, there's a lot of stuff
that ends up not getting said.*
-Catherine Gilbert Murdock,
Dairy Queen

I am lying on the window seat with the blue batik cushion. Outside the bay window the pink plum tree is blowing in the breeze and sunlight is dancing between the leaves. Everything is moving — the air, the light, my heart, my daughter's hand.

Zoey hovers above me, her forehead wrinkled in concentration. She is smoothing my hair away from my face and whispering, "Mommy? Is this better? Do you feel better now? Mommy?"

I feel loved. I feel comforted. But I do not feel better. How do you explain bone-deep, persistent fatigue and pain to a five-year-old? How do you explain fibromyalgia?

Zoey continues to "fix" me. She carries in her toy workbench from the playroom. She chooses the red hammer, the green screwdriver, and inexplicably, a purple hair comb for a baby doll.

"It's okay, Mommy. It's okay. I know what to do." She begins gently to hammer my body — the touch is so soft it feels like the brush of velvet. She screws together my joints moving from my toes up to my ankles, knees, and elbows. She finishes each twist with a wet kiss. She gets out her circular saw and goes to work on my stomach.

She builds me a new body, piece by piece. When she is satisfied with her work, she grabs the comb. She gently detangles all my hair and spreads it out into a fan on the cushion beneath me.

"Mommy," Zoey whispers, "You look just like a mermaid! A pretty, pretty mermaid!" Her face shows so much awe that it takes my breath away.

"I feel like a mermaid," I whisper back.

Zoey holds my hand and we are still for a minute. I imagine myself as a mermaid — floating, and unaware of my body. The water under the ocean is just like the light through the trees — dappled and moving.

I am not my body. I am not pain. I am not fatigue. I just am.

Eyes closed, still touching, I feel Zoey's presence. I feel golden and warm — like I'm cupping the first firefly of summer in my hands.

Chronically Awesome Tips:
Dos and Don'ts —
Talking to Your Kids About Illness

Dos:

- **Talk to them.** Don't put it off. Kids are perceptive and they know when we're not ourselves.

- **Talk to them often.** Once isn't enough. Allow for open dialogue.

- **Include your partner or other important adult.**

- **Pick an appropriate time and space.** Talk in a safe place (like at home) and when you have time. Sit in a space that allows you to see each other's faces and allows your child to have physical contact with you.

- **Keep it simple.** Relay the information in an age appropriate way to your child.

- **Keep it honest.** If you don't know the answer to something, it's okay to say that.

- **Say, "I love you."** Say it often. Make it clear that although your lifestyle may be changing a bit, your love for your child is huge. It doesn't matter how old your kids are, they need to hear this.

- **Tell your child she is not to blame for the illness.** This is especially important for younger kids.

- **Answer questions.** Again, be honest, simple, and direct. Only give the information your child is asking for.

- **Tell your child that she will be taken care of.** Explain that friends, neighbors, grandparents, uncles, etc. may be stepping in at times to help take care of her and things around the house. Let her know that she will never be without support, help, and love.

- **Laugh.** Find something funny and poke fun at yourself and/or the illness. Because there is something silly about it. Really.

- **Find other adults your children can talk to.** Designate a grandparent, aunt, or best friend as another adult the child can go to with questions or concerns. Prep the other adult with the information you have already shared with your child. Invite the other adult to have a conversation with you and your child.

- **Find a way your child can help you if she wants to.** Everyone wants to feel useful. Ask your kid to bring you a glass of water or carry a bag for you.

Don'ts:

- **Don't keep the illness a secret from your child.** Kids are way too smart for this. Include them in an age appropriate way. Not knowing can be a scary thing.

- **Don't tell them about the illness for the first time in the car.** The car does not allow you to see your child's face or hold his hand. The subtext is that you don't really want to talk about it.

- **Don't give too much information at once.** Pay attention to what your child can take in and process. Let the child be the guide of how much and what you tell.

- **Don't assume your child doesn't want to talk about it.** The first time you bring up your illness, your child may be totally silent or change the subject. Tell her the basics of what she needs to know, then allow her time to process. Come back to it.

- **Don't hide all your feelings.** It's okay for your child to know you are sad or mad about your illness. Showing kids a controlled emotion lets them know it's okay to feel those things too. So if you tear up, no worries.

Resources for talking to children about illness:

- Bright Horizons Family Solutions (brighthorizons.com)
- The Child Study Center (aboutourkids.org)
- Wonders and Worries (wondersandworries.org)

Talking to Your Partner:

This is probably not the best way to begin a conversation with one's partner: "Just so you know I have large amounts of internal rage — and it's mostly directed at you." Thankfully, I followed this great conversation starter with, "I know my rage is waaaay disproportionate to what's going on . . . BUT I CAN'T HELP IT." Then I cried.

Actually, my rage was mostly at fibromyalgia. But it's hard to be angry at an illness. Especially when it's your illness. You can't yell at an illness. You can't be passive aggressive to it. You can't wrestle it. You can't walk away from it and slam the door behind you for emphasis.

I was diagnosed with fibromyalgia shortly after Demetri and I got married. It changed everything. It changed our hobbies, our meals, where we lived, our finances, our future. A friend with a chronic illness recently told me, "Once I became sick, it was like each of us had to figure out a whole new relationship with a whole new person. It was starting from scratch." Truer words have never been spoken, my friends.

I was mad, sad, and exhausted. So was Demetri. Demetri is the first to admit that his emotional expression range is that of a teaspoon. Mine is a football field. Demetri expresses his feeling with quiet stoicism. And this sometimes really pisses me off. Although I'm sure my unfiltered, wild, flailing mountain range of intense emotions is not the least bit frustrating for him. Riiiight.

So, there we were, newly married and facing a highly stressful medical crisis. I had to quit my job. We moved from an urban city to a . . . wait for it . . . dairy farm. Demetri went to work during the day and I lay in bed in pain, lost and lonely. I called him a lot with nothing to say. When he came home at night I sometimes didn't get up from the couch.

We didn't know who we were as a couple anymore. We couldn't do the things we were used to doing together: biking, taking long walks, going out to dinner, taking day trips, playing long games of Scrabble. And it was my fault. Sitting was painful. Walking was painful. Being out in public made me exhausted.

Sometimes we cooked together. Sometimes we watched TV. But mostly we stopped talking. Eventually we started

23

yelling. Both of us. It was the first and only time I have heard Demetri yell. He slammed out of the house late at night and walked across the cow pasture until he was swallowed by the darkness. He came back hours later, both of us cried out and scared. And we knew something had to change. We went to couples counseling. We worked on our communication.

It wasn't pretty. And sometimes it still isn't. I yell. Demetri becomes silent. We both fume with anger and pain. But most days we muddle through. Some days we even soar.

Chronically Awesome Tips:
Dos and Don'ts —
Talking to Your Partner About Your Illness

Dos:

- **Include your partner from the beginning**. If possible, have your partner attend some of your medical appointments with you. Once you are diagnosed, make an appointment with your specialist specifically for you and your partner. Use the time to have the specialist explain the diagnosis to your partner. Allow time for you and your partner to voice questions and concerns.

- **Consider couples therapy.** Seriously. Make an appointment right now. You are both under huge amounts of stress. All couples will benefit from a third party providing mediation, insight, and support.

- **Recognize that your partner needs support too.** Yes, your illness is happening to you. But it's also happening to the people who love you. You may not be in a position to offer support because you're dealing with your own stuff. Acknowledge that your partner needs support and give him the time to find it.

24

- **Make a plan.** Work with your partner to decide what your family needs help with and how often. Make it clear that your partner can't take on everything. Help him be okay with accepting help.

- **Be honest and direct.** Tell your partner how you feel and what you need from him. Be specific.

- **Say "I love you."** Even if your partner knows it, say it out loud. Often.

Don'ts:

- **Don't think your relationship will stay the same.** It won't. Chronic illness changes things. It doesn't have to change them for the worse. Get support in maintaining your relationship.

- **Don't take your partner for granted.** Say thank you for the things your partner is doing to support you.

BONUS! Chronically Awesome Tips *for Your Partner*:
Dos and Don'ts —
Talking to Your Chronically Ill Partner

Dos:

- **Believe it.** Your partner has a chronic illness. It's not in her head. She's not making it up. Using hurtful words like "lazy," "crazy," and "weak" don't help.

- **Show up.** Go to doctor's appointments and information sessions.

- **Know about it.** There is no way you can fully

understand what is going on without talking to the doctor. It's fine to do your own research, but ask the doctor where to look for the best information.

- **Accept help.** You can't do everything alone. You shouldn't have to. There are people who love you and want to help. Let them.

- **Remember that you are both doing the best you can.** Acknowledge it.

- **Say, "I love you."** Your partner really really needs to hear this. So much is changing, she needs to hear that your love for her is a constant.

Don'ts:

- **Don't doubt her illness.** If she could make herself better, she would. If you could cure her, you would. But neither of you can fix it, so you have to deal with it.

- **Don't substitute research for talking with the doctor.** There's a lot of info on the web and a lot of it isn't reliable or true. For example, there are sites that say you can cure cancer with only positive thoughts. There's "research" that says chronic fatigue can be cured by jogging. Definitely learn more about your partner's diagnosis, but get your info from trustworthy sites.

- **Don't try to disprove your partner's diagnosis.** If you try hard enough, you'll find that some guy living in his mother's basement published a research study with a sample group of two cats proving fibromyalgia doesn't exist. Showing this to your partner doesn't help. It hurts.

- **Don't try and cure your partner with the latest wonder drug.** If you try hard enough, you'll find that

26

some guy living in his mother's basement published a research study with a sample group of two ferrets proving chronic fatigue syndrome can be cured by this new wonder drug called aspirin. (OMG! Have you heard of it?!) Again, talk to the hand.

• **Don't ignore your own stuff.** You don't have a chronic illness but your world has still been thrown into disarray. It may feel like you've lost your partner, your best friend, your co-parent. You may be going through your own stages of grief. Don't do it alone. Go see a therapist. Deal with your stuff. And yes, it's fair to expect your partner to deal with her stuff.

Resources for more information on health issues:

• Mayo Clinic (mayoclinic.com)
• National Institute of Health (health.nih.gov)
• The New York Times Health Guides (health.nytimes.com)

4

THE OCCASIONAL JERK

Learning to ignore things is one of the
great paths to inner peace.
- Robert J. Sawyer,
Calculating God

One of Zoey's worst tantrums ever took place at Target when she was three years old. She got the shopping cart she wanted, and as she was running around me to stand on the back of the cart, I stopped her. According to her, I stopped her because I'm mean and felt like getting in her way. From my perspective, I saved her young and promising life from getting run over by an elderly man in a motorized cart because I am an awesome mother. The guy had his eyes closed. Seriously.

Phase One of Zoey's tantrum lasted approximately five minutes. Five full minutes of a tantrum is a long, long time, especially when you're in public. However, as I'd already gotten her dressed, out of the house, in and out of the car seat, I decided to press on once she finished screaming. We got the two items I needed and then went to the Christmas section to look at all the decorated trees. I parked the cart at the end of an aisle.

Zoey began screaming, "Nooooo! No! I don't WANT the cart THERE! AAGGGHHHHH!"

Well, excuse me, your majesty. I reached for her hand and said, "Look! A purple tree! Let's go look at it!"

"NO!" She wrenched her hand away from me and careened

29

into a bin full of ornaments. She looked at the ornaments. And I knew what she was thinking: *ammunition.*

I gently but firmly took her by the shoulders and said, "Zoey, you may not pick up those ornaments. You need to get yourself together or we will leave."

She spun away from me again, picked up two plastic ornaments, and threw them on the floor. Then she continued screaming.

I couldn't pick her up – she weighed over 35 pounds – and she knew it. There was no way to remove her from the scene without injuring myself.

"You. Are. In. Time. Out." I hissed. "I will be right over there waiting for you. When you have calmed down we are leaving."

I walked ten feet and sat down on a low shelf that had not yet been stocked with Christmas stuff. Zoey narrowed her eyes, put her hands on her hips, and then fell to the floor.

"Mom-EEEEE!" she wailed. "Mom-EEEEEEEEE!"

A small crowd was gathering. There was pointing. A woman near me asked, "Where is that poor child's mother?"

"I'm right here," I said, raising my hand.

"Oh," she scanned me up and down. "Why doesn't she *do* something? How can she just sit there?!" she stage-whispered to her friend.

Her friend whispered back, "I know. My kids never acted like that."

I thought about explaining. About launching into details about fibromyalgia and telling them that I literally could not pick my daughter up, and even if I could, there was no way I could hold her long enough to get out of the store. But I didn't have the energy. Tears pricked at my eyes.

Zoey continued to wail. "My Mom-EEEE left me!!!!"

"Zoey," I said rather tranquilly, "I'm right here. When you calm down we can go home." After several more minutes of sniveling, whining, and crying, Zoey got up off the floor. I walked over, took her hand, and helped her pick up the ornaments she had thrown. Then we walked out of the store.

Without our purchases. Zoey did not set foot in Target for another nine months.

Maybe I could have mustered the energy to explain fibromyalgia to the two women. Possibly I could have launched into my spiel about fatigue and pain. Conceivably I could have talked about how many parents can just potato-sack their kid back to the car or at least outside. But not me. I have to either intervene or ride it out. And even when I use my best and most amazing interventions, they still only work about half the time. It's not because I'm doing it wrong or because I'm a bad parent (even though it totally feels that way). It's because it's Zoey's job to test limits. And it's my job to hold the boundaries and keep her safe, even when mean judgmental ladies are watching.

I chose not to educate — or flip off — the mean ladies in Target. For starters, I just didn't have the energy. I didn't want to invest time and energy in people I would likely never see again. Plus, I don't think it would have mattered to those women. I think that no matter what I said they would have seen me as a bad mom and Zoey as a bad kid. Those women seemed like the type who don't believe fibromyalgia exists. You know, total jerks.

Sometimes when I see other moms struggling with their kids throwing tantrums in public places I get all smug and think, "Ha! Zoey hasn't done that!" Then I give myself a mind slap and add a single word to my sanctimonious sentence: "*Yet.*" Usually though, I give other parents a smile or word of support. Most often, I go up and say, "I've been there. I just wanted to give you a power mom fist bump. Stay strong!"

One time, when Zoey was blocking the door to the library by gripping one side of the alarm gate with her hands and the other side with her ankles, another mom offered to carry my bag of books to the car. She said, "My kid did that last week." I could have hugged her. Chronic illness or not, being a mom is exhausting. And we never know the full story of what other moms are going through.

31

Chronically Awesome Tips:
How to Deal with Jerks

- **Ask yourself, "Do I actually need to deal with this person?"** If you are never going to see them again, they don't play any kind of role in your life, or if you're not in a position where you have to defend yourself, WALK AWAY. They are not worth your energy or time.

- **Stick to the facts.** As hard as it is, try not to get emotional. Briefly define your illness.

- **Cut it short.** Say what has to be said and end the conversation. It is not your job to convince someone that your illness exists. It is not your job to convince someone of your experience with the illness.

- **Offer to email resources and information.** This is especially useful when you are dealing with someone you have regular contact with, such as a co-worker or another parent at your child's school. It's also a good way to end the conversation yet still provide information.

- **Have clear boundaries.** If this is someone you must deal with, define your boundaries at the beginning of the conversation. Useful phrases include:
  o "I have five minutes to talk you and then I have an appointment to get to."
  o "I don't feel comfortable continuing this conversation now/in front of my children/in this environment."
  o "I'd be happy to have a conversation with you once you have done some background reading on the illness. I will email you some resources."

5

FATIGUE

*My health is the main capital I have
and I want to administer it intelligently.*
- Ernest Hemingway

For me, fatigue is the hardest part of fibromyalgia. It makes me feel like a shadow of myself. The fatigue tends to get all tangled up with depression and pain, to the point where it's all just one big ball of yuckiness that is impossible to sort out. The best way to manage my fatigue, and to some extent my pain, is by very carefully managing my time and energy. Which isn't always possible with a child.

Fatigue can be shaming. I hate for my daughter to see me so tired and weak. I hate to watch my parents lift their own luggage as I stand by and watch. I hate asking a teacher to carry Zoey out to the car when she is still napping at preschool pick-up time. I whisper to myself, "It's okay to need help" and "It's okay not to help." I struggle to remember that there are different ways to be strong.

As we've been told, we have a life-changing chronic illness. So it requires some (drum roll please . . .) life changes. This doesn't have to mean now-your-life-is-really-gonna-suck. But in my experience, not making some crucial changes makes things worse. More fatigue, more pain, and less ability to live the life I want to.

I have six, not-so-awesome, hard-earned Rules of Fatigue:
1. Don't do everything.

2. Use the word "no."
3. Resting might not make it better, but *not* resting will definitely make it worse.
4. Friends should support, not suck.
5. Focus on quality of time, not quantity.
6. Get a theme song.

I am using the word "rules" purposefully. For me, these lessons are not flexible. There is no gray area. If I don't do these things I will have a flare up. Although I know this and I'm writing these rules like I have mastered them, I assure you I have not. Several times each year I throw my hands up and yell, "GAH! Learn the lesson already!" to myself.

Rule #1 - Don't do everything.

Yes, sometimes you will feel guilty about it. I originally wanted to start this paragraph by writing, "Our house isn't exactly dirty, but it's not entirely neat." But this would be a lie. The house is kind of dirty. There are breadcrumbs on the counter and a dried up noodle stuck to the floor under the kitchen table. We did not have noodles last night. Or the night before that. The bathroom has toothpaste and a few strands of hair in the sink. The mirror is streaked with . . . water? Toothpaste? Lotion? Something. The living room is littered with toys, remotes, books, and there's at least one string cheese wrapper and a mostly empty sippy cup under the couch. My bed is not made. It's probably time to wash the sheets. There's a basket of dirty laundry and a basket of clean laundry — none of it folded. There's stuff on the kitchen counter — mail, a My Little Pony, a screwdriver, a shampoo bottle. I'm not ready to go on "Hoarders" or anything, but there's obviously room for improvement.

The reality is that I only have so much energy before the fatigue and pain ramp up and my body begins to crash. Choices must be made. It's a constant balancing act. I have to decide what is most important for my health, for my family, for my friends. Obviously, one thing I often let go of is cleaning. The vacuuming gets done eventually. As does the mopping and the shower scrubbing (by Demetri). I clean off counters and do dishes on a (usually) daily basis. I wipe down the sink and clean the toilet in the bathrooms, uh, periodically. But the other stuff is easy to let go. It'll happen when I have a good energy day. Or Demetri will do it. Or somebody will spill something and at least part of the floor will get wiped up. I've never deeply regretted not having the energy to clean. At least not the way I regret lacking energy for my daughter, my husband, my friends.

My friends are people I don't have to clean for. Or sometimes I clean the first time they come over, and then I say, "Let's be the kind of friends who don't have to clean for each other." This usually goes over well. It's a compliment to be a trusted and loved friend who can come over when things aren't perfect. At least I take it that way.

I have a friend who grew up with a mom with fibromyalgia. After her mom passed away a few years ago her dad hired a house cleaner. He said to my friend, "I wish I had done that when your mom was around. It would have helped her, and me, so much." You know that saying, *if money can fix it, it's not a problem.* If your budget allows you to spend money to have someone clean your house, OHMYGOSH do it. Seriously. Right now.

One may not have to clean every day, but one does have to eat. For me, if I eat like crap I feel like crap. So I have a hyphenated word for you: Crock-Pot. Yes, baby, yes! It works for me on many levels. First of all, I can cook dinner in the morning when I have the most energy. Second, it doesn't use a lot of pots, pans, and utensils, so clean up is easy. Third, IT'S YUMMY. The one downside is the Crock-Pot is heavy. I always have Demetri put it on the counter by the electrical outlet before he goes to work in the morning. I've hurt my neck peeling an orange, so I'm pretty sure I could harm myself by lifting a Crock-Pot.

Another good thing is there are Crock-Pot recipes everywhere. I especially like the blog "A Year of Slow Cooking" (crockpot365.blogspot.com). The woman who writes this blog used her Crock-Pot every day for a year. All her recipes are also gluten-free, so if you're going that route it's super-convenient.

I also have strong beliefs about freezer meals. I hate frozen meals you can buy at the store, but I LOVE the ones I make on my own. I often make double recipes when I have the energy to cook. I freeze the extras. Then, at least once a week, we can eat out of the freezer. Yup, we just defrost some chicken tikka masala or pulled pork or potato soup. TA-DA! A good meal without even trying.

I realize that cooking from a Crock-Pot and not cleaning may not work for everyone. But the key is to find out what you can let go of and, sometimes, what you *have* to let go of. Yard work? Facebook? Laundry? Polishing the silver? Because there is something. There is. In the immortal words of Princess Elsa from *Frozen*, "Let it go! Let it gooooo-oooooo!"

Rule #2 - There's this awesome new word: NO. Use it.

Because I can't do it all, I had to learn to say n-n-n-n-NO. I have to decide how I want or need to use my energy. The n-word has to be used internally and externally. For example, I could browse Facebook and play *Words with Friends* all day long. But it uses mental and physical energy as well as time. I completely shut down my Words with Friends habit and I rarely post on Facebook anymore. I told myself, "No, it's not good for you." And for once, I listened.

I often have to say no to other people. "No, I can't go to Moms' Night Out." "No, I can't help you switch the car seat from the van to the Mustang." "No, we can't meet you at the Science Center." I have to say no to things I know will hurt me, like moving a car seat, as well as no to things I know will take too much energy, like driving downtown and going to the Science Center. This is not to say I will never go to the Science Center. I love to take Zoey places. I just have to do it on a day when someone else can drive and I can take a nap when we get home.

Every day I have to say no to one thing so I can do another. Some days the choices are easy. Well, maybe not easy, but obvious. If I wake up fatigued or in pain, everything is canceled because I have to be able to take care of my daughter. Some days I make compromises, "Yes, I can meet you for lunch, but I can't go to the mall afterwards," or, "We can't go to the playground but we can have a picnic in the yard." Other things involve more difficult choices: "No, I can't watch your child today." "No, I can't bake something for the fundraiser." "No, I can't lift the suitcase for my 65-year-old mother." These choices usually involve disappointing someone else and/or myself. I want to be able to do those things. I should be able to do those things. But often, I can't.

Saying no can be hard. Especially when it's for something we really want to do or to someone we love and genuinely want to help out. But we have to do it. We have to say no. Or else we get really sick and can't take care of ourselves. In these hard situations I find it helpful to make an extra effort to let the person know why I am saying no and I hope that next time I can say yes. Sometimes though, I am too ashamed to explain. I lower my head and plow my way between cubbies in the school hallway, through kids and parents and rain boots thinking, "MOVE, please. I have to get to my car and cry."

Chronically Awesome List:
Ways to Say No

- "No, but thanks for thinking of me."
- "I've got too much on my plate right now. Try me next time!"
- "My time is already committed to _____. But good luck! Let me know how it turns out!"
- "I can't bake a cake, but I can bring paper plates."
- "This time I have to pass."
- "Evenings aren't a good time for me. Can we meet for breakfast instead?"

Rule #3 - Resting might not make it better, but *not* resting will definitely make it worse.

You've probably figured this out already, but ignoring pain, fatigue, and other symptoms isn't the way to go. Powering through doesn't work. There is no cowboying up. Pain does not result in gain. We can't just put on our big girl panties and go. We actually have to (gasp!) listen to our bodies and rest.

This is perhaps the lesson I have to re-learn most often. When I start to feel good and energetic I also tend to get cocky. "Whee! Look at me! I just did three errands in a row! I can totally make dinner tonight!" Or "Hoo-EEE! I just took my daughter to the park! We can totally hit the grocery store on the way home!" My not-listening-to-my-body tell is when I think, "I. AM. A. FORCE of productivity and efficiency. I can do MORE!"

Fibromyalgia snickers and sneers, "Oh? Really? You sure about that?"

It's intoxicating to feel strong, so I ignore the snicker — the tiny tingling of fatigue, the pulsing of pain. Then, WHAM! I get leveled. I am unable to leave the house for days. Lifting Zoey seems like an impossible feat. Heating up soup is a major accomplishment. If I had the energy, I would kick myself for not learning the lesson already.

But here's the real kicker: I can do everything I know I am supposed to do and sometimes the fatigue stays the same or gets worst. I can rest and meditate and cancel plans and do gentle yoga and drink green tea and still feel awful. But *not* resting and taking care of myself causes a flare up 100% of the time. Then I'm benched for days.

Resting definitely ups my chances of feeling better and being able to do what I want to do, but it doesn't guarantee it. There are no guarantees with chronic illness. We all just need to muddle through the best we can, being gentle with ourselves along the way. Because we will miss important things. Things we planned for and we rested for and we waited for. Our hearts will feel a little broken and a little empty. But we will keep going. And maybe the next thing will heal us a little bit. Maybe the next thing will help us feel full.

Rule #4 - Friends should support, not suck.

This is a hard one. Not everyone "gets" chronic illness. To be fair, it is a hard thing to understand fully unless you've experienced it. I've learned to hide pain and fatigue well. Just because I left the house with brushed hair and wearing my nice jeans doesn't mean the pain isn't there. I am happy to explain and answer questions. But if you can't believe that I'm in pain because you don't see a scar or that fatigue is different from being tired — well, it's just not going to work out. Also, if it's going to be high drama when I cancel plans now and then, I'm not the friend for you.

All friendships are give and take. Sometimes I give my friends more than I get. Then we switch. That's what makes it work. I have a friend who once followed me around Target lifting things into my cart for me because there was no way I could lift anything — not even a soup can. I have other friends who wanted me to be able to leave the house so they came over, got Zoey in her car seat, followed me to another location, and took Zoey out of her car seat. All because the bending and lifting wasn't possible for me that day. And on other days, I have cooked for them. Dropped groceries off at their house. Watched their kids. We've vented to each other, consoled each other, and made each other laugh.

When a friend is always in crisis, always stressed, always unhappy, always taking taking taking — I just can't do it. I literally do not have the energy. That's when it gets hard. I have to let her drift away.

Rule #5 - Focus on quality of time, not quantity.

Every day, I try to spend some quality time with Zoey. Sometimes it's an hour, sometimes it's 15 minutes. But for that time, I am totally focused on her and what we are doing together. This practice goes a long way in keeping the two of us connected. It also helps me feel like a good-enough parent on days when I can't do much but lay on the couch. I will cling to the fact that we read together for 15 minutes, Zoey gently patting my hand the whole time. I will console myself with knowing I played Legos for 20 minutes, the two of us building a hang glider for dogs.

Recently, we invented a new game. Tragically (as you will see), the best name I could come up with was Bouncy Ball. The game involves Zoey and me sitting across from each other on the floor with our legs out. We touch our feet together to make a diamond shape. On the count of three we yell, "Bouncy Ball!" and each bounce a ball in the middle of our legs. The goal is to crash the balls together on the up bounce. If your ball gets knocked out of the leg-diamond you lose. If it stays in, you're the winner.

Then this happened:

"Mommy?"

"Yeah?"

"I have a much better name for our game than Bouncy Ball."

"Great! Bouncy Ball isn't such a great name, is it? What's your idea?"

"Vagina Ball!"

[I choke on my own spit due to sudden inhalation]

Zoey continues, "1-2-3 Let's play Vagina Ball!"

I regain the ability to speak. "No. No, we can't name it that. It's . . . it's . . . a personal word . . ."

"I can't wait to go back to school tomorrow! During Show and Tell I'm going to tell everyone how to play the fun game you made up!" And this is a direct quote from my daughter, "Yee-haaw! Vagina Ball!"

Try to do something with your kid every day. Shut your laptop, put down your phone, turn off the TV and just be with them. We may not be able to give them much else on that particular day. But at least we gave them 10 minutes of us. Even if it was while playing Vagina Ball.

Chronically Awesome List:
Things You Can Do with Your Kid While Lying Down

- Read or listen to a book on tape
- Legos
- "Uno" or another card game
- Chess
- Draw
- Do a puzzle (lay on your side on the couch, put the puzzle on a low table in front of you)
- Play-doh (same set-up as a puzzle)
- Play princesses (obviously you are Sleeping Beauty)
- Play with action figures and/or dolls (your knees can be mountains and blankets can be shaped into caves)

Rule #6 - Get a Theme Song.

Seriously. Don't just think about what your theme song would be. Pick one. Download it from iTunes. Put it on a CD, your iPod, your phone. Have it ready to play at strategic locations: by the bed, by the couch, in the car, in the bathroom, wherever you find yourself getting sucked down by the fatigue and pain.

Before I go pick up Zoey from school I often need to play my theme song. I pick her up at 3 p.m., one of the hardest times of the day for me. My body is sluggish and wants to nap. My back and neck pain are gearing up for the afternoon. The last thing I want to do is move.

Time for my theme song!

Currently, it's "Eye of the Tiger" by Survivor. Yup, cliché but true. Even the first few notes make me want to get up and fight. Just like Rocky! By the end of the song I am often slowly and gently shadow-boxing. But still, I am boxing! Sometimes for the first play of the song I have to lie on the floor and just push my fists up at the ceiling.

I put it on repeat and get up eventually. *"Face to face, out in the heat, hangin' tough, stayin' hungry."* EYE OF THE TIGER, BABY! Zoey even has a little boxing/hopping routine she does to the song.

A theme song can't just be any old song. It must be danceable (including car dancing), stand the test of time, and make you feel like you are awesome. My past theme songs included:

- "Little Plastic Castle" by Ani DiFranco
- "Chariots of Fire" (original) by Synthesizer Syndicate
- "Raise Your Glass" by the Glee Cast
- "Dog Days Are Over" by Florence + the Machine
- "Airstream Driver" by Gomez
- "Me and Julio Down by the School Yard" by Paul Simon
- "Here It Goes Again" by Ok Go
- "Float On" by Modest Mouse
- "Closer to Free" by the BoDeans
- "Viva La Vida" by Coldplay
- "Hungry Like the Wolf" by Duran Duran
- "Sing Me a Happy Song" by Melissa Ferrick
- "Comeback Kid" by Brett Dennen
- "Proud Mary" by Tina Turner
- "Laid" by James

You are welcome to steal any of my theme songs. And please email me with your theme song! My family is getting a bit tired of "Eye of the Tiger," so I might need a new one soon.

Chronically Awesome Tips:
How to Fight Fatigue

- **Lower your expectations.** Really. You only have so much energy. Don't waste it cleaning.

- **Only do what *has* to be done.** Dirty dishes eventually have to be washed. But the baseboards? Please.

- **Ask for help**. Your partner might not be clear on what you can and can't do. Divvy up the jobs. Tell him/her you can't push a vacuum.

- **If you can afford a cleaner, DO IT.** Seriously. Take some stress off yourself and your partner.

- **Crock-Pot, baby!** One pot meals that cook while you rest/read/go to the gym? Yes Please!

- **Rest.** Schedule your rest time if you need to. But whatever you do, REST.

- **Say no.** Be choosey. You can only do so much so use your energy in ways that are important to you and your family.

6

HOW TO REST

*I have come to believe
that caring for myself is not self indulgent.
Caring for myself is an act of survival.*
-Audre Lorde

Zoey is two-and-a-half and has been yelling, "I AM NOT SLEEPY!" for the past 24 minutes. I am attempting to sleep on the couch. I need to rest. My body is throbbing, I'm so tired my face hurts, and I am out of patience. Thus far, I am not getting much rest. Instead, I am spying on Zoey with the video monitor and willing her to go to sleep. I watch as she takes a vase filled with water and a flower Demetri gave her last night off her bedside table.[11] She tucks her feet under the sheet and smells her flower with a huge grin on her face. Then she pulls the flower out of the vase and begins twirling it around.

"Aww," I think. "Cute."

Zoey begins sucking on the flower stem. Then nibbling.

"Crunchy," she comments. I quickly Google "gerber daisies" and find them to be non-toxic.

Eat all ya want, kid. I am so not coming up there.

I go about reading my book and settle in on the couch for my rest. I check the monitor one more time. Zoey is standing up in the middle of her bed holding the vase. I watch as she slowly pours all the water out onto her blanket; there is enough

---

[11] Yeah, putting a vase filled with water on a child's bedside table was a totally bad parenting move.

water to make a good-sized puddle.

She begins to jump. I can hear the squishing without the aid of the monitor. Jump. Squish. Jump. Squish. Next she jumps and lands on her butt in the puddle. Jump. Splat. Jump. Splat. I sit, frozen on the couch in horror, unable to look away from the tiny monitor screen.

Then, mid jump, Zoey sees me. I swear she has some freaky super power, looks through the monitor, and sees me. She lands with one more splat, stands up, and peers directly into the camera.

Zoey presses her mouth against the monitor and begins chanting, "Josssss-lynnnnn. Jossssss-Lynnn" And she does it in a creepy frog voice. Zoey continues to chant my name at the rate of 12 times per minute. Yes, I timed it. It's not like I could focus on anything else.

Eventually she gets bored and begins throwing books against her closet door. The board books make a particularly satisfying bang. She has a lot of books so I know I have some time. I begin scrolling through my phone contacts wondering who I can call to get some freaking advice because this situation didn't seem to be covered in any of the parenting books I read. Clearly, this is a HUGE OVERSIGHT by all "parenting experts."

The flower–eating, pool-making, book-throwing "naptime" meant I didn't get any rest. When I don't rest my whole family pays for it. I have less patience, less energy, and less kindness. When I don't rest, I pay for it. My body hurts. I can't do the things I want to do. My relationships with everyone suffer. Especially my relationship with Zoey.

We, the chronically ill, have to rest. As in, we-have-to-rest-right-now-or-the-world-will-end rest. It's often not a choice; it is an immediate need.

Chronically Awesome Tips:
How To Rest with Kids Around

- **Use the magic box with the moving pictures.** I imagined being a mom who didn't allow TV. I now look back at my righteous, pre-parent self and laugh. After Zoey reached the age of two, I began using *PBS Kids* to my advantage. Also, PBS is educational. Like, did you know a squirrel uses its tail for a blanket? Or that the small horns over the Allosaurus' eyes helped it recognize other dinosaurs of its kind? Well then.

- **Use audio books or music.** Some kids get really into this and can sit quietly just listening. My kid was not one of them.

- **Use electronic devices (iPad, iPhone, etc.).** Use whatever will keep your kid safe and entertained for 30 minutes. The iPad has tons of fun and educational apps available to download so your child can up her IQ score while you are resting. For help finding educational apps:
  o Ask your child's teacher. Someone at school should be able to direct you to some good learning apps
  o Ask other parents
  o Try these sites:
    - www.edtechteacher.org
    - www.techlearning.com
    - Search google for "best free educational apps"

- **Use the crib.** If you have a baby, use the crib. Plenty of kids are happy to hang out or snooze in their crib. Unfortunately, my kid was not one of them. But I still used the crib because it's safe. After Zoey was six months old there were times I had to put her in the crib for 10 – 15 minutes and listen to her cry while I whispered to myself, "She's in a safe place. She's in a safe place." I was so spent that I literally could not keep her safe in the house until I got some rest. No one likes to hear her child cry. But a child who is crying out of frustration is preferable to a child who is crying because of, say, a broken arm from falling down the stairs.

- **Make rest time part of the routine.** As Zoey has gotten older, we've called it different things because, tragically, kids eventually outgrow naps. (I know, it's horrible.) So sometimes we have book time, down time, quiet time. Whatever. They are never too old for some form of rest time. Make their room a safe place so you don't have to check on them constantly and let them read books, play dinosaurs on the bed, draw pictures, listen to music. Set a timer for 30 – 60 minutes. You: go rest. This is not a time for Facebook or doing those last few dishes. REST.

- **Give older kids a quiet and engaging activity.** Ideas include: sticker books, legos, puzzles, fun work books (like mazes, word finds, etc.), color by numbers, rubber band loom, finger weaving, dominos, tangrams, paper airplanes, solitaire.

- **Have a "quit time" box.** Put some quiet yet enticing toys/activities in a box. Only allow your child to access these super special awesome toys/games during rest time.

Bonus!

Chronically Awesome List: Toys and Games to Keep Kids Busy

- **Geoboards** by Learning Resources
  $5.00 at amazon.com

- **Eeboo Mosaic Felt Color & Shape Design**
  $16.00 at amazon.com
- **Tangoes Jr.** (magnetic tangrams)
  $20.00 at amazon.com
- **Quercetti Georello Kaleido Gears** (So awesome!)
  $23.00 at amazon.com
- **Funny Faces Reusable Stickers** by Peaceable Kingdom
  $10.00 at amazon.com
- **Educational Insights Play Foam** (no mess)
  $5.00 at amazon.com
- **Pattern Play** by MindWare
  $27.00 at amazon.com
- **Pass the Pigs**
  $10.00 at amazon.com
- **Yahtzee** (travel edition – less likely to lose the dice)
  $17.00 at amazon.com
- **Jenga**
  $10.00 at amazon.com

7

SLEEP

Sleep is that golden chain
that ties health and our bodies together.
-Thomas Dekker

When I imagined being a mother, one of the things I pictured was rocking my baby to sleep at night. I imagined sitting in a glider in the nursery with my daughter's head on my shoulder, both of us softly illuminated by the glow of the moon through the window. Her cheeks lightly flushed. Her mouth, slightly open, exhaling sweet little puffs of baby breath onto my neck while I softly hummed a lullaby. In my imaginings I felt blissful and satisfied.

Before I became a mom, I was so attached to this vision and convinced of its reality, I commented to my BFF, "Sleep deprivation can't be *that* bad." Her daughter was five weeks old at the time. It was probably good we were separated by 650 miles so she didn't have the option of immediately killing me with her bare hands.

I did not once imagine a squirmy, kicky baby who often has more than sweet baby breath coming out of her mouth. Sour spit up and sticky drool did not appear in my fantasies. I did not imagine having to sing "Oh, Come All Ye Faithful," "Rock-a-bye Baby," "My Favorite Things," and all six verses of "American Pie" to get Zoey to go to sleep.

In reality, when I started the last verse of "American Pie" I was an exhausted, strung-out mess. I wondered if I would I ever sleep again. Unfortunately, the answer was not really.

As parents, not only are we in charge of our sleep, but we are also in charge of our child's sleep. We have to tend to them in the night when they are scared or sick. Or when they pee in the bed. Or when they just decide, "Hey, it's 2 a.m.! Now is a good time to have a chat with mom!"

There's a lot of advice out there about sleep. And clearly the standard protocol for good "sleep hygiene" (worst name ever) is not aimed at parents of young children[12] [13]:

Go to bed and get up at the same time every day.

Avoid caffeine.

Sleep in a dark room.

Make sure your room is quiet, peaceful, and uncluttered.

Have a comfortable mattress.

Make sure your room is warm, but not too warm.

Do something restful before bed.

Exercise.

Don't nap.

Most of us will do practically anything to get some good sleep. So we try to do the things on this standard sleep advice list to the best of our ability. Admittedly, our attempts at following this advice often fall short because, well, it's just not possible to ace this list *and* be a parent. Um, I HAVE A CHILD WHO HAS NO CONCEPT OF TIME, let alone "sleep hygiene".

This basic list of sleep advice irks me. Almost every fibromyalgia doctor I have ever seen gave me a version of this list. Each and every one of them handed it to me like they were imparting great wisdom. Plus, it's usually photocopied badly, all crooked and smudged. The fact is that even when all the planets align and I can do everything on the list, I still don't sleep well.

If I'm not going to sleep there's part of me that really wants

---

[12] Deffner, Elisabeth, "Get a Better Night's Sleep," *Fibromyalgia Aware*, Spring 2009: 14.

[13] Longley, Kathy. "My Kingdom for a Good Night's Sleep," reprinted from *FMOnline*, June 21, 2007,
www.fmaware.org/News2ffa1.html?page=NewsArticle&id=5367

to enjoy a cherry Coke and watch a movie about a hot under cover agent or likable criminals. But no. Hell no. That would be too "stimulating." So I don't. I do what I'm supposed to do. I think about how my sleep would be worse if I didn't do the things on the list. But honestly that's not much of a consolation. So, behold! Here are my sleep advice modifications!

Chronically Awesome Tips:
Sleep "Hygiene" Modifications

- **Go to bed and get up at the same time every day. Sort of.** Going to bed and getting up at the same time every day is largely impossible. Several times a month Zoey gets up at 4 a.m. FOR THE DAY. There is no way I am making 4 a.m. my standard wake up time. It's not a bad idea to have a schedule though. During the week I get up at 6:15 a.m. and try to stay awake until 8:30 or 9 p.m. On the weekend, Demetri often gets up with Zoey and I'll sleep in until 7 or 7:30. At night if I'm dragging and hurting I go to bed early. My rising and sleeping times don't vary more than an hour, or maybe two, if I'm really wiped. But it's probably not a great idea to wake up at 7 a.m. then 11 a.m. then 6 a.m. then noon. Even healthy bodies have trouble adjusting to that.

- **Avoid caffeine. Except in the form of chocolate**. This is a hard one for lots of people. Giving up coffee or soda feels like torture. But only for the first week or so. Then our bodies get over it. But giving up chocolate? Well, that would be like living in a world without rainbows and butterflies. I try not to eat a ton of chocolate. And definitely not right before bed. But a small square of chocolate after breakfast? Yes, please!

- **Sleep in a dark room.** So, um, if you're sleeping under a

53

rotating disco ball or a floodlight, don't.

- **Make sure your room is quiet, peaceful, and uncluttered. Or just close your eyes, plug your ears, and walk carefully.** I suck at this one. Quiet? In my room, there's static from the monitor and my husband snores. So I wear earplugs. Unfortunately, the earplugs do not block out either of those noises fully. A room that's peaceful and uncluttered? My room is a den of crap and clutter. There's laundry (clean and dirty) on the floor, and magazines and books cover the floor on both sides of the bed. My dresser is piled high with stray socks, toys that have been confiscated, greeting cards that I can't find a place for and can't throw away, hair ties, and old glasses of water that haven't made it back to the kitchen. I can't get into my closet because the exercise ball and the vacuum are blocking the doorway. All the drawers of my dresser are, inexplicably, open. The wallpaper is what came with the house — shiny, white stripes picked out in 1980 by the 90 year-old woman who lived here before us. The white carpet (also original) is covered in fuzz. Sigh.

- **Have a comfortable mattress.** Sorry, there's no modification for this one. Invest in a good mattress. Your body will thank you for it. I totally ace this one: our mattress rocks. King size TemperPedic, baby!

- **Make sure your room is a comfortable temperature for you.** I like my room to be pleasantly crisp. Demetri refers to this temperature as "freezing," but, you know, semantics.

- **Do something restful before bed. Like going to bed.** By the time dinner is done, the kitchen is cleaned up, stories have been read, and Zoey is finally asleep, I am exhausted. I don't really have the energy to do anything.

Except maybe read or stare blankly at the wall. But, as it turns out, both of those things are restful. So . . . I! Am! Awesome!

- **Exercise.** EXERCISE!!!!! Wooo-Hoo!!! More on this later in the book.

- ~~Don't nap.~~ Whatever. Do what you have to do to get yourself and your kid through the day.

Due to all the poor sleep I've gotten over the past, oh, forever, I now have a healthy fear of going to sleep. So here's some of what I do to lessen my anxiety.

Chronically Awesome Tips:
How Not To Dread Going To Sleep

- **Warm baths** with stuff that smells good.

- **Fabulous pajamas**. I have pajamas and robes that make me smile and make me feel cozy. Target has super cute stuff for cheap.

- **A warm, soft blanket**. I like the micro fleece ones.

- **One good movie**. For those nights when I really can't sleep and I can't stand to stay in bed I get up and watch *Pride and Prejudice*. The one with Keira Knightley and Matthew Macfadyen. I use the remote so I can watch that scene at the end over and over where Mr. Darcy strides across the field in the early morning light with his cloak billowing behind him looking all hot and earnest and. . . hot. The movie is familiar and comforting and not overly stimulating. At least, not in a way that's bad.

- **A cool mist humidifier**. It will keep you from drying out in winter.

- **Warm socks**. I cannot fall asleep if my feet are cold.

- **A good book**. Some people, like sleep doctors, will tell you not to read in bed. They will, in fact, suggest that our beds should only be used for sleeping. I do not subscribe to this theory. Although I am anti TV-in-bedroom I am very much for reading in bed. Reading in bed as part of my bedtime routine helps me relax. It also helps me warm up the bed.

- **Keep your eyes open**. I actually did get this one from a sleep doctor. Apparently, if you wake up in the night and can't fall back asleep it's best to keep your eyes open while lying in bed. I don't know why it works, but it does. The body is easily tricked by reverse psychology. Who knew?

- **Sea-Bands**. These are little bands that have a small plastic ball sewn into them that go over an acupressure point in the wrist. Their primary use is for seasickness and morning sickness. However, a massage therapist told me they also help anxiety and sleep. And they really do. Sea-Bands help me control my anxiety about not sleeping, among other things. I fall asleep more quickly and wake up less often when I wear them to bed. Yes, I do look like I'm from the early 1980s when I wear them but it's dark, no one can see me. You can learn more here: www.sea-band.com. Available at most drug stores.

Go forth and sleep! And if sleeping well is your super power, please email me with instructions. I could use a little help.

8

MEMORY LOSS

The moment when you're like,
WHO THE HELL TOOK MY... Oh... here it is.
- Unknown

One day I pulled into our garage, unloaded the groceries, fixed myself a snack, and began perusing a magazine. I felt capable, efficient, organized. I also felt a little smug. Gosh, I put those groceries away quickly! And look! I was having a healthy snack, an apple and a bit of mozzarella cheese. I was feeling in control. As I began to read my magazine and luxuriate in the stillness of the house, something began to feel wrong. I propped my chin on my hand and began to think, "What had I forgotten? Hmm . . . What was it?"

OH. MY. GOD. I had forgotten my eight-month-old daughter. Zoey was still in her car seat. In the car. In the dark garage. As I ran to retrieve my child from what surely was the most horrific experience of her young life, I had time to think about how I was probably the worst mother on the planet. I committed a monumental parenting fail: I forgot the existence of my daughter. I only have one kid. One! She shouldn't be that hard to keep track of. I remembered to bring in the toilet paper. How could I forget my baby?!

And yet I had. She was asleep when we pulled in. Asleep and quiet. There were a lot of groceries to bring in and then I started making a snack . . . and . . . and . . . and. I burst into the

57

garage, turned on the blinding light, and flung myself up against the car window yelling, "I'm coming Zoooooooooeeeeeeey!!!!"

It's quite possible I startled my child. My child who had been sleeping, but who was now shrieking in alarm at my high-pitched wails and distorted face pressed against the glass. I opened the door, scooped her up, and carried her inside. She stopped crying almost immediately and nuzzled her face into the crook of my neck.

We sat on the couch — me looking for signs of irreparable damage in Zoey's bright eyes and Zoey pulling on my ears and drooling. I'm not saying that Zoey was exactly impressed by my parenting skills, but she didn't seem damaged by them either. Which was lucky.

I once described having fibromyalgia to a friend as humiliating. She was shocked that I would use that word. Memory loss is one of the reasons. My totally non-medical-and-non-research-based theory is our brains are so busy dealing with pain and fatigue that sometimes some of the other stuff gets lost. Getting through the day takes a lot of focus and energy. We can usually remember it's not socially acceptable to yell at the grocery bagger, "Stop touching my apples." On the other hand, remembering to pick up peanut butter at the store doesn't always happen.

It is humiliating and painful to forget about my daughter. It hurts not to be able to remember things that are important to me and to the people I love. I hate being *that mom,* the one who tries to drop her child off at school on a holiday, the one who forgets every single Thursday that it's pizza day, the one who leaves her wallet at home and can't pay for the ice cream. It does nothing for my already fragile self-esteem. No butt and no memory? Jeez, the universe could cut me some slack already.

Let's face it, memory loss stinks. It can make us look like less than our-super-intelligent selves. There's just not a lot of good ways to spin that we forgot our own birthday. Or that we forgot to call a friend back for the third time. At least when we forget why we opened the fridge, we are in our own home, possibly without witnesses.

Don't lose hope. There are several ways memory loss can work for us instead of against us.

Chronically Awesome Tips:
Underlined Ways to Use Memory Loss to Our Advantage[14]

- **Fake memory loss about previous, actual memory loss.** For example:

> Friend: *Remember that time you forgot your own birthday?*
> Us: *No, no I do not remember that.*
> Friend: *Yeah, it was so funny. We were at Starbucks, you forgot about your birthday and . . .*
> Us: *I don't hang out at Starbucks. You must be confusing me with another friend.*
> Friend: *But . . . but . . . I could have sworn it was you.*

    See? See what we have done? We have cleverly caused our friend to question his/her own memory. Thus, erasing the birthday-forgetting incident from our history . . . forever!

- **"Forget" to attend an event.** If there is an event that we are invited to but don't want to attend, memory loss is an excellent aid. This works especially well with obligation events. RSVP to attend the event. Act very excited leading up to the event. Then . . . forget to go. When the host/hostess asks about our no-show status, we let our mouth hang open and our eyes go wide for a second before answering, "No! Oh no! (insert event name here) was yesterday?! I forgot all about it!" Pause,

---

[14] I don't actually use these techniques. But it's fun to imagine . . .

look vaguely stricken and then tap your finger to your temple while saying, "I have such a poor memory . . . it's part of this whole chronic illness thing." If the host/hostess looks like they are the reprimanding type, sigh. Dramatically.

- **"Oh shoot! I forgot them/it at home on the kitchen counter!"** This phrase can be applied to many situations: "Forgot" to get a birthday card for a friend. "Forgot" to bring a dish to a potluck. "Forgot" to bedazzle a mitten for the preschool mitten tree.

It's inevitable that, despite our best efforts, we will forget something that is important to us or someone else. Then we will feel like shit. The good news is that we may forget this feeling later.

Chronically Awesome Tips:
<u>Ethical</u> Ways to Minimize the Effects of Memory Loss

- **Auto-reminders.** Use the auto reminder on your computer and phone. Use them up the wazoo. Google calendar is a great tool because you can send yourself reminders via email or pop-up.

- **Write everything down.** Appointments, grocery lists, names of the new neighbors, when to defrost the chicken, the time of your regular play date.

- **Use calendars.** Google calendar allows you to have several different calendars: one for you, one for your kid, one for your partner. You can view all the calendars at once or only view your own.

Leave yourself post-it notes:

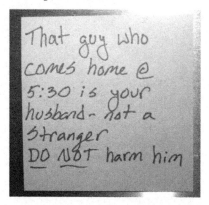

That guy who comes home @ 5:30 is your husband - not a stranger DO NOT harm him

- **Use a blackboard or dry erase board for reminders.** Place it by the door where you exit the house. We use this one from Ikea:

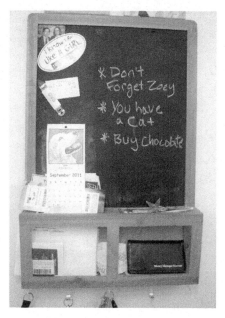

9

THE PIT OF DEPRESSION

Darkness is a path between light and light.[15]
- unknown

Remember when your mom said, "Life isn't fair"? This is what she meant: It is estimated that 1/3 of people with a serious chronic illness also have depression. The exact numbers vary depending on the illness. Up to 71% of us with fibromyalgia have major depression and anxiety disorders.

If you think about all this unfairness though, it makes sense. We are often dealing with some level of pain and fatigue. We don't sleep well. We have to change our lifestyle to be able to function. For some people this means quitting a job, which affects finances and self worth. It can mean dietary changes. Recreational changes. Social adjustments. It puts stress not only on us, but on our family and friends.

In 2011, a survey was published that "revealed the significant impact of pain on daily activities including work, personal relationships and pivotal life decisions."[16] More than 3,000 people with fibromyalgia or another chronic pain condition were surveyed and 9 in 10 felt they were no longer the person they were before they started living with chronic pain:

---

[15] So . . . I have no idea who said this. I remember coming across it in college, but clearly my memory has butchered it to the point that it's unrecognizable. I still like it.
[16] "The Faces of Fibromyalgia." May 2011, *fibrocenter.com*, retrieved August 2, 2012, www.fibrocenter.com/media/Faces_of_Fibromyalgia_Factsheet.pdf .

- 98% of the respondents reported that they had to adapt their daily routine in order to cope with their pain condition;
- 88% had to reduce their physical activity;
- 86% had to adjust household chores;
- 48% approach intimacy with their partner differently;
- 68% of those with children reported that their pain limits their ability to care for their family.

Our lives are changing in ways we never imagined. We aren't able to take care of our kids in the way we want to. We are in physical and emotional pain. So of course we have depression. *Of course.*

Common symptoms of depression include:[17]

- Feeling sad, empty or unhappy
- Outbursts, irritability, frustration, even over small things
- Loss of interest or joy in normal activities, such as sex
- Insomnia or sleeping too much
- Tiredness and lack of energy
- Changes in appetite
- Anxiety, agitation or restlessness
- Slowed thinking, speaking or body movements
- Feelings of worthlessness or guilt, fixating on past failures or blaming yourself for things that are not your responsibility
- Trouble thinking, concentrating, making decisions and remembering things
- Frequent thoughts of death, suicidal thoughts, suicide attempts
- Unexplained physical problems (back pain, headaches)

---

[17] "Symptoms." Depression (Maror Depressive Disorder). *Mayoclinic.org.* Retrieved August 10, 2013. http://www.mayoclinic.org/diseases-conditions/depression/basics/symptoms/con-20032977

One might go so far as to call me The Depression Queen. I'd rather be queen of, say, ice cream and brownies, but I'm told we don't get to pick our titles. I've done my time in the pit. I've been there over and over again. In fact, I've been in the pit of depression very recently.

When I hit the bottom of the pit of depression I know I need to climb up and out. I know I need to reach for the light, but oh mama, it's one hell of a climb. One misstep and I'm back at the bottom, muddy and bruised. Plus, my upper body isn't exactly buff. I have to build up my strength.

Rest. Climb. Rest. Climb. Breathe.

It takes a long time to claw my way up. But when I get there: Oh the warmth of the sun! Oh the sweetness of the grass! And, oh, the fear of falling back in.

Here's the thing with depression: we aren't always either in the pit or out of it. Sometimes we are hanging over the side. Sometimes we are falling. Sometimes we are being pulled in as we are screaming for help and digging our nails into the ground.

The other day I called Tyffany in tears and said, "I'm a crazy sh** a** mother." There was a pause and she said, "Well . . . at least there's no judgment." And I smiled for the first time in days. Perhaps I was *not* being as objective as one can be. Perhaps I was, in fact, being the teeniest bit critical. And dramatic.

But I was also a little bit right. When I feel the pull of the depression, or I'm lying in the dark at the bottom of the pit, patience is something I no longer possess. I am snappish and yelly and, often, just plain mean. I can feel depression reaching out its boney fingers trying to pull me in. I am angry and anxious and needy and lonely all at once. As one might imagine, it takes a toll on Demetri. And Zoey. Which fills me with shame. When I am in the pit of depression I am not the best mom I can be.

Right now I'm teetering on the edge of the pit. I'm in that place where my doubts and judgment and depression and fibromyalgia all meet. My toes are dangling in the darkness and

I'm not yet sure if I will be forced to take a fall. I hate this part — the being-on-the-edge part. I want to just be well or not.

The worst thing is not hitting bottom; it's the ride on the way down. I'm going through the motions and doing the things I know I need to do to feel well: seeing my doctors, asking for help, surrounding myself with people that lift me up and show me the light. And still, STILL I don't know what will happen. Depression is tricky — it can knock you on your ass even when you're doing everything right.

Now I'm in the place of waiting and seeing. Maybe tomorrow will be better. Maybe this afternoon I'll completely lose it. For now, for this moment, I try to be gentle with myself and with my daughter. I'm protecting both of us. We spend hours in the shade of the tree in our front yard making pretend salads with grass and flowers and weeds. And when things get too hard, we watch TV and have a snack. Then maybe we'll have a little dance party. And a nap.

I hope I'll be me again soon. And I know I'll return to being a regular mother instead of ... that other kind of mother.

There are several things that cue me in to ask, "Am I getting depressed?" Some of these things I am not proud of. They're not very, um, cool. I mean, it's not like I start wearing black turtlenecks and writing morose poetry. Nope. Instead, I do things like re-read the entire *Harry Potter* series. I eat chocolate and string cheese at every meal. I don't answer the phone when my best friend calls. I go to bed as soon as it gets dark. I pick fights with my husband and tell him that he wants to leave me.

Then, when things get worse, I stop speaking unless I have to. I wonder if my daughter, who I love so completely, would be better off with a different mother. Finally, I do the most humiliating thing of all: I re-read the *Twilight* series. By this point, I'm pretty well cued in that I'm slipping and sliding into the pit of depression. But often, I still can't quite say it out loud to anyone. It feels too pathetic.

It's humiliating to be back in the pit, to have fallen. Again.

Telling anyone about it would require far too much energy. My body is hurting, my soul feels flattened, and it's all I can do to go through the motions of the day. Sometimes not even that.

From all my time in the pit, I've learned three lessons about depression:

1. Ask for help sooner rather than later.
2. Find a good doctor/therapist.
3. No shame.

I always think I have learned these lessons. "I've got them this time," I'll think, nodding my head wisely. But each and every time I have to re-learn them. I don't know why this is. I'm a fairly smart person. And I have a social work degree, for crying out loud! But there's something about being in the dark pit of depression that makes us lose all sense of reason. It makes us shrink in shame and humiliation. It makes us think we are bad. Really bad. We think we don't deserve anything good: friends, family, sunlight. And we believe with absolute certainty that we are the only person in the world wretched enough to have brought this upon ourselves.

When we are well, we know depression is not our fault. We know if we could have avoided that dark and murky place, we would have. We know that many, many other upstanding citizens have spent time in the pit. And, while we are grateful to feel well, there's also a gentle pull on our sleeve, reminding us that we could go back to the pit at any time. And this makes us afraid.

Here's what scares me the most: that whisper of a thought, just the brush of a feather, that glides through my mind: *What if I drove in front of that bus? What if I wasn't here anymore?* Then I am terrified. I call my husband. I cry. I get help. Right then. I don't wait. I call my doctor. Or have my husband call. I demand to be seen before the end of the day (crying helps with this). I get hooked up with a therapist.

And I get meds.

Medication is a personal choice. I choose it. I'd like to be all whatever-you-choose-is-cool-for-you, but, on this one, I can't. If you are thinking the world may better off without you, if you think your family and friends don't need you, you *need* help. You *deserve* help. You may be able to benefit from medication. And, probably, you need a therapist. NEED. Do it for yourself — get out of the pit faster. The medication doesn't have to be forever. Throw yourself a life-line. You are so worth it.

Sometimes when we are sliding down to the bottom of the pit, we need help. Now. Not tomorrow, not next Wednesday at 2 o'clock. Now. There have been a couple times when my depression got so bad, so suddenly, that I needed medical attention that day. It can be hard to get last minute appointments. Not everyone understands depression can be urgent, even people working in doctor's offices. People may think that because antidepressants usually take four to six weeks to work that it doesn't matter if I see the doctor today or tomorrow.

It matters.

Seeing a doctor, having a prescription in hand, and having a plan to treat the depression is a lifeline. Literally. It makes me feel like I can hold on one more hour, one more day. Having someone listen and see that I need help takes the intensity of the hopelessness down a notch. "Okay," I think. "Maybe I can climb out of the pit one more time. Maybe there's hope." And "maybe" is a huge thing when we're at the bottom of the pit, broken and gasping for breath.

Chronically Awesome Tips:
How to Get a Same-Day Appointment with Your Doctor or Psychiatrist

- **Get a person on the phone.** If you have to leave a message at the office, do so. Then call back every 15 minutes until you reach a live person. Use the answering service if there is one. Ask that a doctor be paged.

- **Say, "I need an appointment today."** Tell whoever is on the phone you feel hopeless and overwhelmed and you're not sure what will happen. If you've had even the teeniest thought of maybe, possibly hurting yourself, SAY IT. This is not the time to downplay your symptoms. If you are denied an appointment . . .

- **Kindly but firmly demand to speak to your doctor.** Do NOT leave a message. Instead, say, "Please get Dr. Smith on the phone. I'll hold until she is available." Talking to a nurse or physician's assistant may also be helpful. If you are still denied an appointment . . .

- **Drive to the office and say that you need to be seen.** Bring a book. Sniffle and blow your nose loudly in the waiting room. Go up to the desk every 20 minutes or so and kindly remind them that you're there. They should fit you in.

If You Think You Might Hurt Yourself:

- **Call your doctor or therapist.** If your doctor's office does not say, "Come in right now," take yourself to the nearest emergency room.

- **Call an ambulance.** If you can't get yourself to the ER or shouldn't be driving, call 9-1-1. Do it. There are people in the world who love you. One day soon you will love yourself again.

- **Call someone.** If you can't bring yourself to call an ambulance, call anyone. Your neighbor, your friend, your dentist, it doesn't matter. Get someone on the phone. Tell them what's going on. Ask them to drive you to the ER. Ask them to call an ambulance.

What To Do at the Doctor's Office or ER:

- **Be honest.** Even though it's painful to say our deepest fears and secrets out loud, do it. Get the help you need. Trust me, you are not the first person or the last person to feel useless, empty, and like a drag on everyone you know.

- **Get a referral for a psychiatrist and a therapist.** Your doctor may be willing to prescribe meds for you. That's great. Start them. Then follow up with a psychiatrist. Medications can be very tricky. They take a while to work, they potentially have a lot of side effects, and it can take some time to find the right medication/s for you. Psychiatrists are the experts at prescribing medications for depression, anxiety, etc. Use them.

- **Directly tell your doctor what you need.** If you don't know what you need, say it. It's okay to ugly-cry and blubber out, "I . . . feel . . . so . . . bad. I just need hel . . . helll . . . help." It's also okay just to cry for a while. I once went through an entire box of tissues in about 15 minutes. My doctor took it very well. If you're at the ER, don't even worry about what the doctor or nurse is thinking. Trust me, those people have seen everything.

Other Treatment Options: Transcranial Magnetic Stimulation

And yet sometimes medication doesn't work. Or it only kind of works. Or it has terrible side effects. Years ago when I first began taking antidepressants, they worked. True, there were some side effects, but they were manageable. A headache here and there. A bit of nausea. Occasional night sweats. I could deal with the side effects because I felt better. I even eventually felt good.

As years went by, I tapered off the medication, did okay, got depressed, and was put back on the medication. While in graduate school, my usual meds stopped working. I didn't feel like driving in front of a bus, but mostly because it would take too much energy. Getting out of bed felt like running a marathon. I rarely thought about the future because it somehow seemed there wouldn't be one. When I looked ahead everything was gray and heavy.

So my psychiatrist started changing up my medications. Eight years later I had been on over 25 different types of medication for depression. I had gotten used to headaches, drenching night sweats, and the inability to have an orgasm. I was taking ibuprofen on a regular basis, sleeping in my moisture wicking running clothes in an effort to get the cold sweat away from my skin, and, you know, *faking*.

I went to see a fibromyalgia specialist who said, "I think if we could get either the depression or the fibromyalgia under control your life would be a lot better." Fair point. He recommended I look into transcranial magnetic stimulation (TMS) — a non-invasive procedure with little to no side effects that uses magnets to stimulate electrical currents in the brain. The idea is that the electrical currents will change brain activity, allow new pathways to form, and improve the symptoms of depression. TMS was approved by the FDA in 2008 and is most effective on people with treatment resistant (doesn't respond well to medication) depression.[18] To be clear, TMS is NOT electroconvulsive therapy (ECT) or "shock therapy" in which seizures are electrically induced in patients who are anesthetized. ECT, though often effective, is an invasive procedure with potentially serious side effects, such as memory loss.

---

[18] Melkerson, MN. "Special Premarket 510(k) Notification for NeuroStar TMS Therapy System for Major Depressive Disorder" (pdf). Food and Drug Administration. December 16, 2008.
http://www.accessdata.fda.gov/cdrh_docs/pdf8/K083538.pdf (7 January, 2013).

People who have not experienced depression, the ineffectiveness of medication, and intense side effects would likely respond to a procedure that involves their brain by running away. Or shrieking, "Not my brain!!!" I, on the other hand, responded with giving the advising doctor a fist bump, "My brain! What a great idea!"

I went home and energetically researched TMS. Mayo Clinic. NIH. McLean Hospital. Johns Hopkins. No side effects? No pain? Works best on people who are not responsive to medication? TMS was clearly invented just for me. I was totally in. I linked my family to informative articles. I expressed my enthusiasm with an excess of exclamation points.

My family was not as excited as I was. Whereas I saw the potential for help, they saw the potential for harm. My dad took me out for Thai food and said with his eyes glassy, "I just don't want you to have any more problems than you already do." I could feel my dad's fear. And his love. But all I could think was, *If I don't try this, I'm going to be like this forever. I'm not sure I can do this forever.* My mom and Demetri also expressed their concern. Everyone was coming to me to make them feel better about the treatment.

Finally, I exploded, "It's not my job to make you feel better about something that is happening to me. I sent you articles. You all have access to the Internet. I can't make you feel better about this. I'm doing it. If you don't like it, fine. But I don't want to hear about it anymore." And then I cried. I was angry at my family for not seeing how this was a lifeline for me. I was angry because depression is like parenthood — it's almost impossible to understand unless you've been through it. And I so badly wanted to be understood.

I went to the initial TMS appointment on my own. I filled out depression questionnaires. I met with a neurologist and a psychiatrist. I asked too many questions and took pages of notes. I booked my first appointment.

My mom came with me for the first treatment. I think she knew my feelings were hurt by the family's lack of enthusiasm. Also, I think she wanted to be there to hold my hand if my brain exploded or I had a seizure. Moms are like that. To be honest, I was nervous. Brains are pretty important and when you add an electrical current to it, even one stimulated by something innocuous like magnets, well, it should give one pause.

My mom and I sat in the office flipping through *People* and making snide comments about the rich and semi-famous. Every few pages my mom handed me another Hershey Kiss, the silver foil flashing a sweet promise of hope. Then a man, a young man, came out to greet us. He was dressed professionally in khakis and a button down and had kind eyes, but there was something about his walk that worried me. His walk was . . . buoyant. This clearly was a young person who had not yet been beaten down by life or depression and fully believed in goodness. I am also a person who believes in goodness, but somehow my walk isn't so light.

Zach, the buoyant young man, clearly knew his stuff. He answered all our questions clearly and thoroughly. He made some appropriate jokes. He put us at ease. Finally, my suspicions got the best of me. "Do you have a certification in TMS or something? Did you graduate from college? What are your qualifications?" At the time, it seemed important that a person shooting electrical currents through my brain have at least a four-year college degree. And Zach did. Plus, lots of experience administering TMS.

Then it was time to begin. I sat in a cushy chair while Zach put a swim cap on my head, took some cranial measurements, and made some marks on the swim cap with fruity smelling markers. Zach clearly had lots of practice taking people seriously with swim caps on because he didn't mock me once. Zach held the magnetic coil that would be placed on my head in his hand and said he would run it once so I could hear what it sounded like. In the space of two seconds there were forty clicks that sounded like a really fast, really loud wood pecker. Next Zach tested the coil on my arm so I could see what it felt like. It was a quick vibrating tingle.

Then he did it on my brain. It made my nose feel like a

73

tuning fork. And that was it. The treatment consisted of 40 applications of the coil, so every 30 seconds I got two seconds of nose vibration. By the end, I had a slight headache and was ravenously hungry. Those side effects I can live with.

TMS may be for you. Or not. But if you suffer from treatment resistant depression, take the time to find out.

10

STRESS

*Behind every stressful thought is the desire
for things to be other than they are.*
-Toni Bernhard,
How To Be Sick

A few years ago, I had a major fibromyalgia flare-up just before
Christmas. As it happened, it was the first Christmas we were
hosting family at our house. Also, it was Zoey's second
Christmas. Her first Christmas, I reasoned, she definitely
wouldn't remember. But the second Christmas? Well. That
would likely be burned into her 20-month-old brain forever. I
planned the menu weeks ahead of time, bought special plates
with elves on them, and tied our Christmas tree to the banister
so it wouldn't fall over on anyone. I decorated. I planned out a
timeline for the night — when we would eat, when Santa
would come, when Zoey would open her first present. I made
Demetri go into the forest and cut down real evergreen
branches so we could make a wreath. I may have even done an
Excel spreadsheet that was color coded.

Two days before Christmas, just when all the baking and
setting up was scheduled to begin, I crashed. Hard. I couldn't
lift a can of cranberry sauce. I couldn't lift my daughter. I rarely
got out of bed. I couldn't do any of the prep work I had
planned. After much counseling and then threatening from my
mom, I did the hardest and smartest thing — I let it all go. I
got the heck out of the way and let my family take over. I'm

not even sure I washed my hair on Christmas Eve. I just showed up, descending from the bedroom into my own living room. Which actually was a big accomplishment.

It was great — my best Christmas ever. Seriously. I was relaxed. I was grateful just to be there. I soaked up the glee on Zoey's face as Pop-Pop lifted her up to touch the star on the top of the tree. I leaned against Demetri's shoulder and ate Christmas cookies. I watched my mom watch her granddaughter with amazing tenderness. I felt happy, something I'm not sure I would have felt if I had stuck to my color-coded schedule.

Chronic illness and life in general seem to be affected negatively by stress.[19] As in stress tends to exacerbate everything — pain, fatigue, poor sleep, depression, low energy. Besides using my energy wisely, saying no, and investing in supportive friends, there are a few more things that may help with stress reduction. Chiropractic work, massage therapy, acupuncture, meditation, and talk therapy are all thought to help with stress reduction.

Lucky you! I have tried all of these things and I am going to tell you about it. As a side note, all of these things can be somewhat expensive (unless your insurance covers it;), so you may have to decide which is the most helpful. I use chiropractic work, massage therapy, and talk therapy on a regular basis. I use acupuncture on and off, depending on my needs.

Chiropractic Work

It took me an entire year to work up the courage to go a chiropractor. I had this image in my mind that the main job of a chiropractor was to spin my head around *Exorcist*-style. Frankly, I was afraid my neck would get broken. Or my back. I thought that having a broken neck and/or back might

---

[19] "Fibromyalgia (FMS)." *Arthritis.org.* Accessed February 13, 2014.
http://www.arthritis.org/conditions-treatments/disease-center/fibromyalgia-fms/

possibly make things worse for me. Also, I imagined a chiropractic doctor to be a big, burly dude who spoke in monosyllables — sort of like a caveman. His giant muscles would squeak as he broke my neck, "Heh. Oops. Me muscles big. You broke."

But I had so much pain and was feeling so helpless and just needed help help help. I found a chiropractor who came highly recommended from a trusted source and — joy! She was a petite woman who radiated kindness. She did a mix of chiropractic work, acupressure, and energy work. And she was gentle. I explained my fears to her — about her twisting my head around — and she understood. She told me that I needed to be comfortable with everything she did or she wouldn't do it. There was stuff I wasn't comfortable with at first. And she was okay with that.

Here's generally what happens when one goes to see a chiropractor. You go and sit in a waiting room — likely they will have good magazines, free water, and little candies at the front desk. The chiropractor will take you back into a private room where there will be a cross between a massage table and a doctor's table. Your first visit will be 30 minutes or longer. The doctor will explain what chiropractic work is and how it works. Then she will go over your health history with you and you will get to ask questions and express concerns. The chiropractor will examine your back (you may have to do different things like lie on the table or stand). Some places take x-rays. Likely, the doctor will gently press on your back, measure your leg lengths, and gently press along your neck. Then the doctor will explain how she thinks chiropractic work can benefit you and will suggest certain types of adjustments. Some chiropractors will have you lie on a table with heating pads on your back and neck. Next, if you are comfortable, you might get adjusted. Sometimes during an adjustment you will hear a quiet pop from your back or neck.

Some of you may start to panic and hyperventilate and say, "My back! Did you break it?!?!?!"

The chiropractor will look at you with patience and extreme

kindness and say, "No, it's not broken. That popping sound is just air releasing from your joints."

You might feel stupid but don't, because know that someone who came before you said the same thing. That same person may have even cried out of nervousness.

How to Find a Good Chiropractor:

- **Get a referral from a trusted source** (A friend who exhibits good judgment in other areas of her life = a reliable source. A friend who listens to country music and eats marmite = an unreliable source).

- **Call several chiropractic offices and ask to speak to the chiropractor.** Ask him/her if they have treated patients with your illness before and how their treatment of those patients differs from those patients without a chronic illness. Ask them what they know about your illness. If either (a) the chiropractor won't talk to you on the phone and insists you come into the office, or (b) the chiropractor doesn't answer the question thoroughly and honestly, DO NOT GO THERE UNDER ANY CIRCUMSTANCES. I don't care how close it is to your house or that there's free parking.

- **Note how you feel when you go into the office.** Is it comfortable? Is the staff friendly? Do you feel like you're in a good place? If not, fake a stomachache and get the hell out.

- **Note how you feel when talking with the doctor.** Does she make you feel comfortable and safe? Does the doctor seem knowledgeable? Do you feel like you're being talked into things that you're not comfortable with? Does the doctor look at you when speaking? Does it seem like you're just another part to be fixed on a conveyor belt or is the doctor really hearing and seeing you? Remember: Just because you are in the presence of a chiropractor does not obligate you to get examined, x-rayed, or adjusted. Yes, you can just walk out. Trust me, I have and nothing bad happens. Well, except for the people in ski masks with baseball bats chasing you . . .

Three Ways to Spot a Bad Chiropractor:
1. **He/she won't talk to you on the phone** before coming in for your first appointment. Okay so this may not be the best marker for judging a good chiropractor. But in my opinion if the person isn't willing to spend a few minutes answering questions on the phone, he probably isn't invested in making sure his clients are comfortable and informed.
2. **The office does not have private rooms for adjustment.** I once went into an office where all adjustments took place in the middle of a busy waiting room. Um . . . no thanks!
3. **The chiropractor doesn't go over your health history** before beginning an exam. When you are seeing a doctor for the first time, she should always always always review your health history.

Does Chiropractic Work Hurt?
This is a tricky question. I can only answer how it is for me. The truth is that sometimes it kind of hurts. Or more like aches intensely. But only for a few seconds. That ache is more than worth it for the hours or days of relief that come with the adjustment. When I first started getting chiropractic adjustments, I went in three times a week. The intensity was tolerable or I would not have been able to go back. The first time I got adjusted, I was incredibly tired afterwards. So plan your first appointment when you can go home and rest following the adjustment. For the first few weeks, I was occasionally a bit sore the next day. But this kind of soreness was so much more preferable to the pain I had been experiencing on a daily basis. The soreness was actually a relief. Every single time I have gone to my chiropractor, I have walked out feeling much better than when I walked in.

Massage Therapy/Body Work

Probably if you're a regular kind of person, the idea of getting a massage is awesome. Relaxing. But once I was diagnosed with fibromyalgia my response became more along the lines of, "Wait. What? Someone is going to *touch* me? Like, on my *body*? I DON'T THINK SO." I knew that, in theory, massage could help me. Even though it took me a long time to try it as a healing modality, I totally screwed it up. My first mistake was that I went to see a massage person at my gym because they were having a special. I may be stereotyping here, but I have learned that massage therapists that work at gyms are (a) generally recent graduates, and (b) think all their clients are super athletes and will benefit from deeeeeeep tissue massage. This particular massage therapist kept telling me, "You'll feel great tomorrow! This is the perfect pressure — I totally learned this in school! Of course you trust me, right?" What I should have said was, "Um . . . I just met you. I do not trust you. GET YOUR HANDS OFF ME AND I MEAN NOW, LADY!" What I actually said was, "Um . . . well. Ok. I guess."

I now know that just because I'm lying naked on someone's massage table, she has access to my body, and her massage school certificate hangs on the wall (even if it's in a frame!), it does not mean that I have to trust her. Within 90 minutes of leaving the massage-at-the-gym I was in intense pain. And out 60 bucks.

In another massage experience (one that I would like you to note has never been repeated), the massage therapist "massaged the waste through the intestines" for "optimal detoxification." So yeah, this lady I had just met massaged poo through my body. As I was leaving she said, "You might want to go right home. Or at least be somewhere there's a bathroom." I never went back to her again. Not that the technique was bad per se, I personally just found it weird, uncomfortable, and anxiety provoking.

In case you've never had a massage before, here's what to expect: First you will meet with the massage therapist while you are fully clothed to fill out some paperwork and go over your health history. The therapist should be doing more listening than talking. Tell her if it's your first massage and be honest about any massage anxieties you may have. Eventually, the therapist will leave so you can get undressed and situated on the table. Before she leaves she will tell you to lay face down or face up. It's okay to leave on your underwear if you feel more comfortable that way. I also sometimes leave on my socks so my feet don't get cold. Lie on the table and cover yourself with the sheet. The therapist should knock before re-entering the room. Once the therapist comes back in, she should tell you a bit about how she is going to start and ask you to comment on the pressure. Feel free to comment on the pressure often and at any time during the massage. The masseuse will only know what works for you if you tell her.

How to Find a Good Massage Therapist:
- **Again, a referral from a trusted source is optimal.** BUT realize that if you get a referral from a friend who runs marathons and gets sports massages every week, you and your friend may be looking for very different things in a massage therapist.

- **Insist on communicating with the massage therapist before booking an appointment.** Ask her if she has worked with people with _____ (insert your chronic illness here) before. When she says yes, push a little bit harder. For example, "Great! Tell me what you know about fibromyalgia . . ." I once had someone reply to this, "Um, hold on. Let me get my phone so I can Google it." This is what is known as a red flag. The massage therapist should be able to give me a thorough definition of fibromyalgia and demonstrate an understanding that deep tissue massage may not be the most effective thing. Hopefully, she will talk about working with you to find the optimal healing experience.

- **The best massage therapists do NOT work at gyms or spas** (in my humble opinion). I have found my best massage therapists at my chiropractors' offices or integrative health centers.

Five Ways to Spot a Bad Massage Therapist:
1. **The therapist asks you to undress in front of her.** You should be given privacy and respect.
2. **The massage therapist offers to have sex with you.** No. Just no. This is what is known as "crossing a boundary."
3. **She doesn't ask, "Is this pressure ok?" repeatedly.** You want a massage therapist who is constantly checking in with you and is open to feedback.
4. **You don't feel comfortable telling your massage therapist that something hurts or is not what you want.** Your massage therapist should be open and responsive to your feedback.
5. **Any touch feels invasive or inappropriate**.

Does Massage Therapy/Body Work Hurt?

Truthfully, it might. I know, I know, you want to hear that there's at least one thing that is all about relaxing and feeling good. But this isn't it. At least for me. I love how I feel after the massage. But reminding my muscles to unclench and getting some of the knots out doesn't always feel so good while it's happening. My massage therapist works with me and the pain never goes above a 5 on a scale of 1 - 10. The pain is also not constant; there's a lot of the massage that feels great. Plus, my massage therapist has a tinkly little fountain and gentle music playing in the massage space so that's nice.

Acupuncture

Acupuncture is the insertion of needles into the body at specific points called acupuncture points. Yes, this one involves needles so you can imagine how long it took me to work up the courage to go. I insisted on talking to the acupuncturist on the phone before going in. (Are you sensing a theme?) Luckily, he was very reassuring. He told me it didn't hurt and that I would have no ill effects afterwards.

I went. I lay on a table and let some guy I'd never met before stick needles all over my body. Then he shut me in a darkened room with quiet music and . . . I fell asleep. Well, first my body turned in to a pool of relaxed mushiness and then I feel asleep.

It. Was. Awesome.

I tried acupuncture for several months. It helped me a lot with stress and anxiety but it didn't have a huge impact on my fibromyalgia symptoms. However, I know several people who credit acupuncture with completely alleviating their fibro pain. So, hey, it could be worth it.

About the needles — they're not like sewing needles. Yes, I did imagine being stuck with sewing needles. They're incredibly thin and flexible. After they are used once, they are then thrown out. I especially liked having them stuck in my ears — totally relaxing.

How to Find a Good Acupuncturist:
- **Referral!!!!**
- **Call and talk to the acupuncturist first.** Share your concerns. If he is reassuring and able to explain what he will do, that's good.
- **Check out his website** — do they have your illness listed as something they treat?

Five Ways to Spot a Bad Acupuncturist:
1. **He won't talk to you on the phone** before coming in.
2. **When you tell him your concerns he responds with, "Just trust me."** You just met him. Of course you don't trust him.
3. **The office is dirty or the acupuncture room is not comfortable and relaxing.** Acupuncture is supposed to be relaxing and healing. If the office is prohibiting those feelings, go somewhere else.
4. **He doesn't explain what he's doing before he does it.** In my opinion, a good acupuncturist (or a good doctor) will

explain what he's doing before he does it. Treatment goals and modalities should not be a surprise.

5. **He doesn't go over your medical history** and discuss your goals for acupuncture *with* you.

Does Acupuncture Hurt?

Not usually. Occasionally there would be a needle that would pinch a bit as it was going in. Generally I never felt the needles going in. For me, acupuncture time was nap time; I found it very relaxing.

Talk Therapy

So, I sense that you're feeling ambivalent about therapy. Can you tell me more about that? Ha, ha. Just kidding! That was just a little therapist humor because I was a practicing therapist – until fibromyalgia struck. No, really, it's true. I have an advanced degree and everything. You know what else? I have sat on both sides of the couch so to speak. In fact, I would never see a therapist that has not been through therapy him/herself. After all, if my therapist hasn't dealt with her own crap (yup, that's the technical term) how in the world is she going to help me with mine? I also would dump a therapist who says the first two lines of this paragraph in seriousness.

I have used therapists many many times in my life, often for depression, but several times specifically for fibromyalgia. The first time was when I was first diagnosed. My husband and I had gotten married about two months before the diagnosis and started couples therapy one month after the diagnosis. Nope, we weren't on the verge of divorce. We just felt like we needed a little bit of support communicating about all the sudden stress and life changes that we had not been expecting. Going to therapy took the edge off. Suddenly there wasn't so much yelling (me), crying (me), and overwhelmed silences (him). Win!

Then about two years ago, I went and saw a fibromyalgia medical specialist. This specialist told me that I had fibromyalgia. Again. And you know what? It threw me for a loop. It was baaad. I had sort of kind of hoped the specialist would tell me to buck up! That I was a wimp! That there was nothing wrong with me so go out and lift things and travel and do, you know, regular stuff! But no. Instead I was offered more pain meds and badly photocopied Thera-Band exercises.

Somehow it was like being diagnosed for the first time all over again. I was angry and confused and so, so tired. I felt like a drag on my family and friends. I felt like a bad mother, a bad wife, a bad person. I think my heart cracked just a little bit. This was for real. My life was going to be different than I imagined it. At the time, this crack in my heart felt so raw and damaging. But it's healed a little bit and now I see it as one of those cracks that's a sign of use and of love.

I worked with a therapist who had a halo of grey hair and kind eyes. In her office she had a foot-high statue of Quan Yin, the goddess of compassion. The statue was white marble, and my therapist had strewn the area in front of Quan Yin with pink flower petals and a line of tea light candles. I often stared at the statue instead of at my therapist — especially when I was crying. Both Quan Yin and my therapist sat and listened while I cried about how unworthy I was, how totally valueless. Eventually, I began to feel better. I began to be in motion — moving forward, moving on, moving out of the stuckness and sadness. Now I have a small statue of Quan Yin by my bed. It's made out of a magical substance that glows blue in the dark. When I can't sleep at night, I stare at the Goddess of Compassion and am comforted by her blue light and by the knowledge that she has seen me at my worst and still sits by me in non-judgment.

How to Find a Good Therapist:
- **Again: referral, referral, referral.** If you are unable to get a referral, Psychology Today has a reasonably good database of therapists, and allows you to search by geographic location, specialty, gender, etc. (http://therapists.psychologytoday.com)

- **The first therapist you go to may not be a good fit.** If the therapist makes you feel scared, shamed, or guilty — ditch her. A good therapist will make you feel comfortable, supported, and accepted.

- **Not liking your therapist and not liking what she says are two different things.** A good therapist will occasionally challenge you to think about things in a new way; she may initially offer some insights that are not immediately comfortable to you because they are not familiar. However, you should still feel supported and safe during this process. If you don't, run out the door and try someone else. You should never ever feel unsafe in a therapy session.

- **It's important to have a therapist that is working with you where you are at right now.** If you feel your therapist is constantly dragging you ahead or behind, it's not going to work.

Six Ways to Spot a Bad Therapist:
1. **She or the office smells like alcohol or marijuana. Um,** red flag!
2. **Your therapist offers to have sex with you.** Again, boundaries.
3. **The therapist talks a lot about him/herself.** Therapy is about you. You you you.
4. **The therapist checks her phone/email during a session.** Her complete attention should be on you. In the rare instance that it's not, she should explain why. For example, "I have a patient who was admitted to the hospital this morning. I am expecting a call from the ER doctor. I apologize, but I'll have to excuse myself for just a minute to take it."
5. **The therapist takes a lot of notes to avoid eye contact.** Many therapists do take notes. They should also be able to look at you from time to time.
6. **The therapist can't remember anything about you from one session to the next.** A therapist should be able to

retain information about you from one session to the next. If she doesn't know your name, find someone else.

Does Talk Therapy Hurt?
Not physically. Unless your therapist has an uncomfortable chair. But it can be emotionally hard at times. You will be talking about some painful and difficult things. Often, after you get the stuff out and off your chest you will feel better, lighter. You may even feel more in control. Not every session is hard. Some sessions will be great and energizing. It's all about working through things — which often involves a mix of emotions.

Bonus section!!
Chronically Awesome List:
Ways to get out of booking another appointment if you don't like the practitioner

- "I need to check my calendar at home before setting up the next appointment."
- "I need to see when my babysitter is next available."
- "I need to check with my insurance company about how many sessions are covered."
- "This isn't a good fit for me."

Mindfulness Meditation
Regular practice of mindfulness meditation is a useful tool in helping people cope with pain, depression, anxiety, and improve their quality of life[20]. Mindfulness meditation involves sitting, being present in the moment, and not judging yourself

---

20 . "Mindfulness Meditation: A New Treatment For Fibromyalgia?." *Sciencedaily.com*, accessed February 13, 2014.
www.sciencedaily.com/releases/2007/08/070805134742.htm

or your thoughts. Often people will focus on their breath or a mantra while practicing mindfulness.

I have only recently begun practicing meditation and I find it to be very helpful and very hard. It is challenging for me to just be with myself and my body, even for a few minutes. I always lie down to meditate. My body gets twisted and knotted with pain if I try to sit. When I try to meditate on my own, it goes something like this:

> Deep breath . . .OK, I can do this . . . Focus on the breath . . . Ahhh . . . Oh, wait, I need to relax my stomach . . . Ahhh . . . my back hurts . . . I think I'll lean against the wall . . . I really like brownies . . . brownies with chocolate frosting . . . Wait, my mind is wandering . . . Come back to the breath . . . Ahhh . . . Weird, I can feel my breath in my left arm . . . And in my right hip . . . I wonder if the cat is staring at me . . . Maybe I should open my eyes and check . . . No, no I shouldn't . . . FOCUS ON THE BREATH . . . Ahhh . . . my breath feels swirly in my chest . . . is swirly a word . . . probably . . . Vanilla ice cream is actually really good . . . My mind is wandering . . . Come back to the breath . . . Ahhh . . . I wonder if I went to a mindfulness retreat if the Buddhist monk would yell at me because I'm so bad at mindfulness . . . That would be embarrassing . . . But I'm not sure a Buddhist monk would be allowed to do that . . . If I was yelled at I would have to leave because that wouldn't be a very accepting environment . . . Why am I even thinking about this? . . . Focus on the breath . . . Ahhh . . . I wonder how long I've been doing this . . . This might be the longest I have ever meditated . . . Yay me . . . Focus on the breath . . . I should probably get a real meditation cushion since I'm doing so well at this . . . I deserve a meditation cushion . . . Maybe they make them in purple . . . GAH! Come back to the breath . . . Ahhh . . .

Then I check the clock. It's been four minutes. I shut my

eyes again and try and go for another six minutes. It's sort of painful. Which is why I now use guided meditations.

Apparently, after several months when I am a more practiced meditator, it will get easier. Or, at the very least, one's body and mind get used to it. I'm not there yet.

The point of all this is we need to pay attention to and manage our stress. We're parents, we'll never be stress free. But illness wraps another layer of stress around our minds and bodies. We need to pay attention and take action.

Other Mindfulness Meditation Resources:
- *A Path with Heart* by Jack Kornfield
- *Guided Meditation: Six Essential Practices to Cultivate Love, Awareness, and Wisdom* by Jack Kornfield
- *How to Be Sick: A Buddhist Inspired Guide for the Chronically Ill and Their Caregivers* by Toni Bernhard
- *Mindfulness Meditation: Nine Guided Practices to Awaken Presence and Open Your Heart* by Tara Brach, PhD
- Insight Timer – I love love love this app. It's free and offers over 60 different guided meditations and a self timer options. It's on my phone which makes it super convenient.

11

EXERCISE

The only bad workout
is the one that didn't happen.
- Unknown

Yes, we get it. We're supposed to exercise.[21] Exercise and stretch.[22] I have enough badly photocopied Thera-Band regimens from doctors to fill, oh, just hypothetically, a trashcan. Note to doctors: if you want me to do something give it to me like you mean it. Make sure the photocopy is clear, fits on the page, and isn't crooked. Your inability to work a copy machine doesn't exactly inspire confidence. A crookedly copied and smudged sheet makes me not take you seriously. In fact, I get this image of you rummaging through your files muttering, "Hmm. What can I give her to make it look like I know what I'm doing? Ah ha! A *photocopy*!

I have tried most forms of exercise available/suggested. Some went better than others. This chapter of the book is less advice-y and more embarrassing-y than previous chapters. Embarrassing for me, not you. My hope is that these less than stellar exercise stories will convince you that it's okay to try new things. It's okay to be slow. It's okay to fall off various

---

[21] Bennett, Robert. "Newly Diagnosed Patient." Fmaware.org, accessed February 14, 2014. http://www.fmaware.org/ PageServer0bbc.html? pagename=fibromyalgia_overview

[22] Dupree Jones, Kim and Janice Holt Hoffman, "Exercise and Chronic Pain: Opening the Therapeutic Window, *Functional*, Volume 1, Number 4, January-February 2006. http://www.myalgia. com/Exercise/ICAA_Functionalu_Vol4_1.pdf

pieces of gym equipment. Most of this stuff won't happen to you. Probably. But if it does, know you are not the first.

But before we get to the stories, a bit of general advice.

Chronically Awesome Tips:
General Exercise Advice

- **Start slow.** Even if you were a gym rat in your pre-chronic-illness life, this still applies to you. Ease your body in to the new routine. Be consistent and gentle. You need to see how your body responds before you can amp up the activity.

- **Set reasonable goals.** Reasonable: "I will walk for 15 minutes four days this week." Unreasonable: "I'm going to run five miles every day this week even if it makes me puke!" Remember, your ultimate goal is to find a form of exercise that you enjoy and you can do on a regular basis. Anything involving pain and puking needs be crossed off the list.

- **Borrow DVDs from the library.** This allows you to try something like yoga or Pilates from the comfort and privacy of your living room. No walk of shame out of the exercise class! If you can't do the exercises or just don't like it, just turn off the DVD. The downside is no teacher to ensure that you are doing the exercises safely and correctly.

- **Find a buddy.** Find a walking buddy, or a gym partner, or a yoga friend. Having an exercise partner helps us be accountable and consistent.

- **Try new things.** Take a chance and try the new gentle yoga class, water aerobics, or the spin class. The worst thing that happens is you walk out. If you hate the class or it's too much stress on your body, pretend you got an urgent text on your phone and walk out with an air of importance. So you tried something new and it didn't work. You tried! You win!

Swimming

When I was first diagnosed with fibromyalgia, my doctor insisted I take up swimming. I bought a real swimsuit (as in a Speedo, not a tankini with a skirt), earplugs, and goggles. I looked fast. Or I would have looked fast if I didn't have so much non-aerodynamic jiggly fat. But I went to the pool anyway. I got in. I swam a few laps. Read as: I swam partial laps, stood in the pool, and gasped for breath. I was passed by senior citizens. I kept swimming. I was asked by the life guard to get out of the swim lane so the "swimmers" could "swim." I retreated to the hot tub where, despite my body being sausaged into a bright turquoise swimsuit, I was mistakenly identified as "Hank" by a gang of old men. Hank was their 75-year-old buddy that they were expecting to join them in "the tub" (as they called it). This did not lift my spirits. Although I did feel marginally better when they told me they couldn't wear their glasses for tubbing. One guy made a point of making sure I knew he was really, really blind without them.

I went back to the pool six times. My shoulder and neck pain got worse. And worse. I also began to feel worse about myself. How could I not even swim one lap? How come it wasn't getting easier? How come my no-butt looked like cottage cheese? I hated every minute in the pool. So I stopped swimming; it just wasn't the right thing for me. The tubbing was pretty good though. Especially since the gaggle of old men had stopped calling me Hank.

Biking

After I refused to continue swimming, my doctor recommended biking. I again refused. Here's why: for our honeymoon, my husband and I drove our bikes 950 miles to Maine. My bike was brand new — a surprise pre-wedding present from Demetri. We had one specific ride we wanted to do and we were pumped. The Day of the Bike Ride dawned and we threw our gear into the car feeling all bikey and hip. We reached our destination, put on our helmets, and saddled up. We went about 100 yards and I fell into a ditch. We were not off-road biking. We had been on a path. A wide path. Yet I hit the ditch. I smacked my head/helmet and got gravel in my face and hands. It was super sexy. I tried to be brave. We had just gotten married and I suspected that my new husband didn't know the full extent of my wimpishness. Yet. The braveness lasted about four seconds at which point I looked up at Demetri and blubbered, "I think I'm going to cry now."

My fear of biking was born.

Demetri walked our bikes back to the car while I sniffled along at his side. My new husband picked gravel out of my hands and chin with tweezers. He fed me pop-overs. And he bought me biking gloves. Three years later I was finally able to get back on the bike and ride a block. Not around the block. Just a block. I was a quaking nervous wreck the whole way and kept yelling, "OH MY GOD! A CAR! A CAR!" or "Give me SPACE! You're going to CRASH into me!" for the entire 30 seconds.

Then my doctor convinced me to try a *stationary* bike. Totally genius, right? I screwed up my courage and went to a spinning/cycling class. It was awesome. First of all, spinning classes take place in a dark room. Which means no one can really see what you're doing, unless you fall off your bike. Not that I would know anything about that. Second of all, you are in charge of adjusting the resistance level on your bike and there is no way for other people to tell what resistance you are at. This means that the twenty-year-old next to you with the perfect butt that actually fits on the bike seat will never know what level you're at. After class you can say to her, "Wow, class was kind of easy today, I was at a nine the whole time," and you can watch her mouth form a pursed little frown that will contribute to the wrinkles she will get in about ten years. Also, they play really good, fun music and you feel like a bad ass. Especially when you stand up and pedal.

Yoga

I'm sitting on my purple yoga mat waiting for class to start. I'm sure I'll feel Zen and flexible any second — I'm in a high ceilinged room with bamboo floors, scented candles, and soft music. How could I not? Because I am always early everywhere, I am the first person to stake a claim on floor space. In the back. The way back.

I watch the other students come in. I notice they seem to be giving me a wide berth. My first thought is to wonder if I smell. But no, I showered and class hasn't even started yet. Then I begin to sense that perhaps my sweatpants and t-shirt with holes in the armpit were not the best fashion choices for class. The other women are wearing tight fitting, black yoga pants and tiny yoga tanks with spaghetti straps and racer backs. Also, makeup. Most of the other women have on lipstick, eyeliner, etc. I don't think I've ever even worn eyeliner. My lipstick? It's called Chapstick. So before class has even started I'm feeling a little betrayed. I expected to be in class with a bunch of touchy-feely overly welcoming hippie types. Or at the very least, I expected to be in class with people who didn't care what I wore.

Then the instructor bounces in. Literally. There is no other way to say it: The woman has clearly had a boob job. Also, she is hot. Like H-O-T-T-T. She is wearing a very short skirt. And, I kid you not, a tube top. Yeah, yeah I just said I wanted to be in class with people who didn't judge me for what I wore but . . . but . . . it's a TUBE TOP. With NOTHING underneath. No sports bra. No bra bra. I am immediately anxious that my instructor is going to fall out of her top during class. This is not going to help me be Zen. In fact, it's going to make me highly anxious about a wardrobe malfunction. If I were truly Zen I would focus my thoughts inward. I would be a pool of calmness. But I'm a BEGINNER and this is asking too much.

Then the instructor opens her mouth, "Ya'll," she chirped, "I just got my hair done! Do you like the blond?" Most of the students fall all over themselves saying how "great" and "natural" her hair looks. As I said, Yoga Barbie (which I will now call her out of cynicism and jealousy) is hot. Yes, she has fake boobs. And fake hair. And is wearing significant amounts of make-up. But she also has a six pack, rock hard thighs, and an ass that probably looks really good in jeans, or naked.

She begins to settle us in for class. We sit, eyes closed, and breathe deeply while Yoga Barbie chirps at us. "Center yourself, focus your attentions inward," she instructs. I try but all I can think about is Yoga Barbie's boobs. Are they heavy? Does she, perhaps, have back problems? Are they ever cumbersome?

"Be here, now, in this practice." Yoga Barbie breathes loudly and deeply and I wonder if that's how she sounds during sex.

"Yoga is about doing the best practice you can do. It's about who we are on the inside. The *inside*."

I can't help it, I snort back a laugh. I'm pretty sure the people closest to me mistake the snort for deep breathing — at least no one shoots me a dirty look. I peek open one eye and see Yoga Barbie adjusting her tube top in the mirror. And I see that I am not the only one watching her. Ha! Ha-HA! I am not the only non-looking-inward-boob-focused-mediocre-pseudo-yogi.

Then we begin sun salutations. We reach up, arch back, and go into downward dog. And there, hanging before the whole class, like a hypnotizing pendulum (except there are two of them) are Yoga Barbie's breasts. Contained, only in the loosest possible sense, by the tube top.

Look away, I tell myself. *Just. Look. Away.* But I can't. They are hypnotizing — every single person in the room is staring at them. We are five minutes into class and I already have an anxiety stomachache about when it is going to happen. If the boobs come out early in class, how will we make it through to the end of class? Will we pretend nothing happened? Will she go get another shirt? Or . . . Oh. My. God . . . What if it happens *more than once*? My eyes snap down to my mat.

"Okay. Nine more sun salutations to go," chirps Yoga Barbie.

Somehow, 54 minutes later I make it to the end of class. I do not feel relaxed. I feel skittish and I have a crick in my neck.

Since then I have done yoga with several other teachers. Some of the experiences have been good. But they're not as fun to write about. I recommend gentle yoga. The classes are more low-key and the teacher and students tend to understand chronic illness. Yoga is a great thing for many people. It's not my favorite form of exercise or meditation. Partly because I have never been able to touch my toes. But also because classes are expensive and I seem to get greater pain relief from cardio. I enjoy yoga best when I can do it in the privacy of my living room. You know, so I can wear a tube top.

Pilates

Wikipedia describes Pilates as:

"a body conditioning routine that helps build flexibility and long, lean muscles, strength and endurance in the legs, abdominals, arms, hips, and back. It puts emphasis on spinal and pelvic alignment, breathing to relieve stress and allow adequate oxygen flow to muscles, developing a strong core or center (tones abdominals while strengthening the back), and improving coordination and balance. Pilates' flexible system allows for different exercises to be modified in

97

range of difficulty from beginning to advanced. Intensity can be increased over time as the body conditions and adapts to the exercises. No muscle group is under or over trained. It enhances core strength and brings increased reach, flexibility, sure-footedness and agility."[23]

I did not try Pilates until very recently. I had been doing yoga in my living room but it was aggravating my knee and wrists. I got several Pilates DVDs from the library thinking that maybe strengthening my core would help my whole body. Basically, I hoped it would help me feel like less of a weakling.

At first, it made me feel like more of a weakling. I couldn't do some of the exercises because my "power house" was weak. But then it got stronger. My stomach looked flatter in the mirror! I felt like I had some muscle! I could do The Teaser! When I first started I had some soreness in my stomach muscles. It was the good kind of sore, not the fibromyalgia kind of sore. Now I do 25 minutes of Pilates every other day. I feel better in my body and I feel better about my body.

Running

Many a doctor steered me away from running saying it was "too much," "too high impact." But you know what? Running is one of the few things that helps me — really helps me.

I should point out that I am a slow runner. I don't feel slow. I feel rather spry when I run. But, apparently, I am slow. Very slow. One weekend Demetri and I were driving along Storrow Drive in Boston — right on that stretch of road by the river where there's a paved trail, beautiful grass, and a great view of the city. There were also about a zillion walkers, runners, and bikers. We were stopped at a light and an older runner shuffled and dragged his way past us. He was tired, out of breath, and not so graceful. *Ha!* I thought, *Ha! At least I'm faster than that guy!* Except that I accidentally said it out loud.

[23] "Pilates." *Wikipedia.org*. http://en.wikipedia.org/wiki/Pilates

Like, in front of other people. But thankfully only in front of Demetri, who already knows I'm the tiniest bit crazy, and Zoey, who was sleeping. But still. Thinking crazy, selfish, overly competitive thoughts is one thing; saying them is another.

Demetri, assuming I was talking to him, sort of paused, made a soft humming sound, and said, "Well . . ."

I whipped my head around from the window and the pitifully slow runner to look at the profile of my husband. My husband who was very intently looking at the traffic light.

"WHAT?! I'm as slow as that eighty-year-old guy?! That one right there?" I pointed out the window. We both looked. Mr. Eighty-Year-Old-Slow-Runner-Guy was now stopped in the grass bent over, one hand on his knee, one hand clutching his chest.

"Whoa. Is he okay?" Demetri asked.

"I'm sure he's fine. Stop avoiding the question. Am I as slow as that guy?"

"Well, it's hard for me to tell exactly. We're in a car and everything . . ."

"We're in a car THAT'S NOT MOVING! So . . . so . . . so you're trying to tell me," I slumped back into my seat, "I'm as slow as that guy."

Part of me knew it was true. I know, at least on some level, that I am a slow runner. I know that some people can walk faster than I run. Some people can even hula-hoop while walking faster than I run. The Silver Sneakers, the over 70 running club at the Y, has a few members that can take me.

The thing is, I don't feel slow. When I run, I feel fast. Swift. Dare I say, lithe. Even after someone passes me, blows by me, crushes me. As soon as they are out of sight, which usually happens pretty quickly, I am back to feeling like an Olympic runner prancing nimbly down the path. I am happy to be the fastest and most graceful runner in sight. And happy that fast is a feeling, much like beautiful is, that can be kept in my head and in my heart.

Strength Training

I recently signed myself up for regular PT sessions. And for once, it doesn't mean physical therapy. Nope. I am locked in to a year of personal training sessions. You know, as if I was just a normal, non-fibromyalgia person. *La di da! Look at me! I'm just going to lift some weights! Whee!*

Except, I suspect, my fitness goals are rather different than most other people at the gym. When my trainer asked me during our first session what my fitness goals are, I said I have two: (1) To be able to lift a bag of groceries without pain and without injuring myself, and (2) To be able to kayak for 10 minutes without serious pain that lasts for days. The trainer, whom I will call Ronnie because that's not his name, nodded his head sagely. Then he said, "We can do that." Points for Ronnie!

So my first session with Ronnie went kind of like this:

(Ronnie demonstrates how to use a machine. Then I try.)

Me: *Whoa! I'm awesome! This is a lot of weight!*

Ronnie: *Don't forget to breathe.*

Me: *But I'm lifting things! With my arms!*

Ronnie: *Focus on your form. Keep the elbows in.*

Me: *I've already done five and my arms aren't shaking!*

Ronnie: *You're doing great!*

Me: *I didn't know I even had this much muscle!*

(Ronnie looks at his clipboard, almost like he wants to avoid eye contact)

Me: *How much weight am I lifting?*

Ronnie: *Don't worry about the weight, just focus on your form.*

Me: *But look! I'm lifting something! How much? What, 20 or 30 pounds?*

Ronnie: *Well, technically you're not lifting anything…*

Then he went into some long-winded explanation of how the machine has no weight on it and a counterbalance so I'm not even lifting the bar-thing and how he just wants me to get used to the machine and proper form blah blah blah. It took me a minute to get over the shock that lifting nothing really felt like lifting *something*. I decided I could feel bad about my lack of muscle or I could feel . . . not bad.

Me: *But I look like I'm lifting something, right?*

Ronnie agreed. So that's what we're going with: looking like I'm lifting something. And it's better than where I was before: forlornly looking at things I couldn't lift. Soon I will *actually* be lifting something. That's right, baby, I've got nowhere to go but up!

Thera-Bands

Thera-Bands! Oh, how I want to love thee! In case you don't know what Thera-Bands are, they're kind of like giant rubber bands that come in different colors that represent different resistance levels. They are gentler than free weights and can be used for strength training. Thera-bands are good because (a) they can be used at home, and (b) they can be used for much more than exercise. I recommend having a session with a personal trainer or a physical therapist to get some good Thera-Band exercises and to make sure you do the movements correctly. But once you have that down, oh baby oh! you don't have to leave the house to exercise. This is especially useful when one feels so crappy that even the idea of getting dressed and stepping outside is nauseating. Often times when we feel like this our bodies still need gentle exercising and stretching. I know, it seems impossible. But you can do it.

On the down side, Thera-Bands are boring. You have to stand there looking at your wall or staring at your ceiling while you do repetitive movements. For me, this is one exercise regimen that often gets kicked to the back of the closet. I would much rather do exercises on a balance ball or do Pilates. Thera-Bands just aren't lively enough for me.

Because I dislike Thera-Bands, I have come up with multiple uses for them. They can be used as a sling-shot. They can be used to keep your three year-old out of the snack drawer. (I recommend using them on the snack drawer, not the child.) A Thera-Band can also be tied around your head while playing Ninja Warrior. It can be used as a streamer for interpretive dance. Or, in a pinch, as a belt. It can also be used to tie a Christmas tree to the railing of the stairs so it doesn't tip over. Ah, versatility!

Exercise/Body Ball

Yes, I have fallen off my exercise ball. It was only because someone (Hi Kelly!) told me it was possible to balance on top of it on my knees while not holding on to anything. It's so not possible. Well, maybe if you're in the circus. But still, I love that blue ball. It's fun to bounce on, it feels great to stretch on, and it's gentle. Believe it or not, you can work your entire body using this one ball. You can also use it for massage. Like, on your back, shoulders, hips, and butt. I have the Valeo Body Ball which came with a poster on how to use it. I have also worked with my physical therapist and chiropractor on good stretching and strengthening exercises with the exercise ball.

When I'm having a horrible fibromyalgia day, even just sitting on the ball for a few minutes helps. It engages core muscles, improves balance, and helps relieve back pain. But only if you don't try to stand on it.

Chronically Awesome Tips:
How to Go to a New Exercise Class and Not Feel Like an Idiot[24]

- **Get to class early.** But don't go in. Wait until someone else goes in first, then follow them and do what they do. If they get a yoga mat, a block, and a blanket, do the same thing.

- **Sit in the back.** If you're not sure where the back is,

---

[24] I can help you not feel like an idiot, but you may feel like a weakling. Everyone does at the first few classes. Everyone.

which often happens in yoga rooms, go for the side by a wall. Also sit near the door. It's your first class, and when you've had enough you may want to slip out. It's dangerous to try and walk through a room of people doing sun salutations or doing jumps on bikes.

- **Introduce yourself to the teacher.** Explain it's your first class. This is especially important in a spin class. The teacher will help you get set up on the bike. Trust me, if you try and do it on your own without having any experience with stationary bikes, bad/embarrassing things will happen.

- **Always always ALWAYS bring a bottle of water and a towel.** You may sweat up a storm and you'll want something to wipe it on other than your shirt. A shirt can only do so much.

- **Stop if you need to.** If you feel embarrassed about needing a break, stop and "stretch." This is perfectly respectable. You can even sit and stretch. All you have to do is put your legs out in front of you and reach. It's also perfectly respectable to just stop. Everyone's done it at one time or another. If you feel you need an excuse: redo your pony-tail, adjust your shoe lace, make sure your water bottle isn't leaking, refold your towel, fix your earring, blink a lot as if you have something in your eye. But whatever you do, take a break when you need it.

- **Bring a friend with you.** Bribe her if necessary. Friends make us feel more confident, even when neither of us has any idea what's going on.

12

DOCTORS

If we cannot change the way things are,
the skill of life becomes learning how to feel deep love
and care for what is flowing through our fingers,
even while letting go.
- Andrew Olendzki

Dear Doctor,

I know you have received years of medical training. I see you graduated from an Ivy League school. No, I didn't know the frame is real gold. Very nice. I see you have a family — the picture on the beach of all of you in faded jeans and crisp white shirts is lovely. Uh, sure, now that you mention it, I am vaguely impressed by the stethoscope hanging around your neck.

I wanted to give you a bit of advice. You know, from the patient's point of view.

- **Make sure everyone in the office has empathy.** Lock them all in a room and make them watch *Beaches* or *The Notebook*. Anyone who doesn't cry is fired. Including you.

- **Learn how to work a copy machine.** When you give me photocopies that are crooked and blurry it makes me wonder how you got into college, let alone med school.

- **If a patient is crying, offer her a tissue.** "Offering a tissue" does not mean run out of the room and send in a nurse with a tissue.

- **Apologize if you are running late.** We may not be doctors, but we are people. We have our own families, jobs, schedules that should not be less important than yours. I'm okay waiting for you. Especially if you take your time with me and don't rush me.

- **Introduce yourself and make eye contact with your patient.** Graduating from medical school does not excuse bad manners.

- **Believe your patient.** If you don't, refer her to someone who will. Patients have the right to be taken seriously.

- **Have good magazines.** Sitting can be painful for a lot of us after oh, three minutes, so we like to be distracted by gossip, news, fashion, cooking, etc.

- **It's okay to make jokes.** Just not at our expense.

- **Be reachable.** Set aside time for phone or brief email contact with your patients.

- **It's okay to say you don't know.** It's okay to say you will look into it. It's okay to say you will confer with a colleague. We will respect you for saying this. We will not respect you for making stuff up, for blaming us, or for ignoring us.

- **When you give someone a new diagnosis, tell her about it.** Give her written information. Then give her a few minutes to sit in the room without you there to think and look at the info. Come back, sit, and ask your patient what questions you can answer. This gives us time to process.

- **Remember I am doing my best with what I have.** I'll try and remember the same about you.

- **Hand out chocolate.** You know how kids get lollipops and stickers after an appointment? Yeah. Do that with chocolate.

Sincerely,
Your Patient

P.S. I'll try not to be snarky about your gilded diploma. And stethoscope. And family photograph.

It takes most people years to get a diagnosis of fibromyalgia. I was lucky. It only took me six weeks and five different doctors to get a diagnosis. This was partly because my primary care doctor loved mysteries and was really pushing her colleagues to figure it out. And partly because I was lucky and got connected with good doctors right away.

Aside from a couple of amazingly positive experiences, my interactions with doctors have been less than stellar. In general, doctors seem to blow me off once they hear "fibromyalgia." Before the "–ia" is even out of mouth they ask, "Are you in counseling?" I explain that I have had counseling where I've talked about and dealt with having a chronic illness. I've been in counseling for depression, relationship issues, and stress management. The doctors tap a writing utensil impatiently.

"But have you gone to therapy for the fibromyalgia? To get rid of the pain?" I explain to them that therapy does not "cure" fibromyalgia. When they keep pressuring me about therapy I ask if there's someone else in the practice I can work with. Or, alternately, I hold back tears and ask them to please check me for strep throat, which is what I'm there for in the first place.

Some doctors seem to blame everything on fibromyalgia and miss other diagnoses. For example, I had horrible knee pain for over a year that prevented me from running. I was told again and again that my fibromyalgia was presenting in a new way. Well, as it turns out, I had a torn lateral meniscus and needed knee surgery.

I have spent a lot of years building up resentments towards doctors and their lack of empathy, communication skills, and sincerity. Sometimes I have rage towards a doctor before I even meet him. I am certain he will waste my time. Often I am right. Or I wait months to see a specialist. She's great but her staff isn't. I have no access to the actual doctor after the appointment and am left to navigate medication doses, side effects, and new symptoms with an incompetent staff. With one particular specialist, I was going back and forth with his assistant about medications. After sending her several emails and trying multiple medications to alleviate pain, terrible side effects, and worsening sleep, she wrote me an email that said, in its entirety: "wanna try something else?"

There are so many things wrong with that response. First off, and this is coming from someone who is by no means a grammarian, "wanna" isn't a word. The first letter in a sentence should be capitalized. I felt like I was emailing with a twelve year old. It would have been appropriate, and dare I say professional, for her to acknowledge the difficulties I was having and then, perhaps, list some alternative medications, what they do and why they might be more effective. The email made me feel disrespected, unimportant, and like I was not receiving adequate care.

About a year ago, I was on a waiting list to see a fibromyalgia specialist for over six months. When the day of the appointment finally arrived, I spent the entire 60 minute drive to the hospital thinking, *Don't hate the doctor before you get there. He's going to be great. It won't be a waste of time.*

I waited 45 minutes past my scheduled time in an over-heated waiting room without any magazines. I was taken back to his office and made to stand (there were no chairs except the one behind his desk) for another 15 minutes until he came in.

Then an overly tanned, squat man who looked like a former wrestler gone to seed breezed into the office with a takeout cup of Starbucks coffee and sat at his desk. He shuffled papers while I stood there awkwardly. I wasn't even sure he knew I was there.

I shifted my purse on my shoulder and cleared my throat. "Hi?" I ventured.

He didn't look up. "Well. What are you doing here?" Except it wasn't a friendly so-tell-me-why-you're-here-today-and-how-I-can-help-you. It was a sharp bark along the lines of why-the-heck-are-you-in-my-office-taking-up-my-time?

I was so shocked I thought there must be a misunderstanding. "Um, you're Dr. Hill, right? The fibromyalgia doctor?"

"Obviously."

I would like to point out that Dr. Hill was not wearing a nametag and there was not a nameplate on his office door so it wasn't exactly obvious.

"I have fibromyalgia," I squeaked out.

"So?" he replied without looking up.

"Well . . . I was hoping you could help me with that." I toed the ground nervously.

"How am I supposed to help?" Again, he didn't look up.

I wanted to yell, "Could you make this ANY harder for me, you pig-headed jerk?" But instead I shuffled my feet because I was STILL STANDING and said, "Do you have my chart? I filled out your five pages of paperwork that says why I'm here."

He sighed, closed his eyes, and pinched the bridge of his nose. Clearly, I was the most tiresome patient he had ever encountered. His fingers seemed swollen and his wedding ring appeared to be linking two fleshy sausages together. "I don't have time for this. Tell me why you're here and what you expect me to do, otherwise I can't help you."

I had three simultaneous thoughts: (1) Ohmygawd. This

man has a wife, (2) Ew. Does he actually touch her with those sausage hands? and (3) I waited six months for this freaking appointment, this man needs to be less of an ass and more of a doctor.

I planted my feet, took a big breath and said a more diplomatic version of number three, "I waited six months for this appointment, please stop giving me such a hard time. You're the doctor, so please act like it."

And, bingo! The man made eye contact. He did an exam. And yes, he touched me with the sausage hands. They were cold and rubbery on my neck. It was not a great moment. After 90 minutes with Dr. Hill, The Amazing Fibromyalgia Doctor, he diagnosed me with . . . tennis elbow. Not fibromyalgia *and* tennis elbow. Just tennis elbow.

I vibrated and crackled with rage. "How does tennis elbow explain all my pain and fatigue?"

Dr. Hill shrugged and said, "It doesn't."

Then my rage, as it often does, turned to tears. I would much rather be a fearsome rage goddess who expresses her anger eloquently, or at least intelligibly, instead of a limp, whimpering child who can't speak because odd and ugly sounds will come out of her shaking mouth. It was humiliating to cry in front of Sausage Hands.

I gathered my things and managed to hiss between shaky breaths, "This is the worst —" breath "experience I have ever had —" breath "with a doctor." Stifled sob "I hope —" sniffle "you are one day treated —" gulp and sniffle "how you treat your patients." And I left with my head held sort-of high.

Until Dr. Hill called after me, "You dropped your mitten." And I had to go back into his office and pick it up off the floor.

I know. Don't you just want to hug me after that?

Chronically Awesome Tips:
How to Find a Good Doctor

- **Referral.** If you know someone who has a chronic illness, go to that person first. A referral from someone who is mostly well is not the same as a referral from someone who is often unwell.

- **Call up the office.** Tell whoever answers the phone your primary diagnoses and anything specific you are looking for in a doctor and/or doctor's office (i.e. a female practitioner, a doctor who communicates via email, a lab in the same building). Often the front desk staff will be honest and tell you if they have a doctor who might be a good fit.

- **Make a 'Prospective Patient' Appointment.** This is an appointment where you can interview the doctor. Come with a list of questions. For example:
  o Do you work with patients with fibromyalgia?
  o What do you generally recommend as treatment?
  o When you refer a patient to another doctor, how do you choose that doctor? Is it someone who you have worked with before?
  o Is it possible to get a same day appointment?
  o Are you willing to communicate with my other providers (i.e. therapist and fibro specialist) by phone or by email on a regular basis?
  o Will I see you or a nurse practitioner most often?

- **Speak to more than one doctor.** I know — this is a pain and takes a lot of energy. But it's worth it.

When we moved to Boston I found the most amazing nurse practitioner without even trying. Taryn (a) believes that fibromyalgia is real and, (b) can make eye contact with me while talking about it. Taryn is smart, on-time, and wears cute shoes. I've been seeing Taryn for about two years. A few months ago, I decided I trusted Taryn enough to give her my list of daily symptoms (25+) and a list of all past medications (20+). I had never trusted a medical professional enough to do this before.

She didn't back towards the door or ask me about therapy. She responded as I hoped she would: she was willing to look for any other underlying causes for my fibromyalgia symptoms, do tests to rule out other illnesses, and refer me to other doctors and specialists to help me feel my best. Of course, I'd had many of the tests done six years before when first diagnosed, but Taryn was willing to do them again to see if anything had changed. She was willing to look for Zebras.

I did multiple blood tests, urine tests, and cardiac tests. Taryn sent me to an orthopedist for back, neck, and hand pain. She recommended a massage therapist. She found me a new fibromyalgia specialist.

I arrived at my follow-up visit with Taryn feeling hopeful, almost buoyant, that maybe something else was wrong. Not like cancer wrong. More like low iron level wrong. In other words, something easily fixed. Something that could be treated. In the first few seconds of the visit, I knew something was off. Taryn wasn't looking at me much. She kept jiggling her foot. She took a big breath.

"Well . . . we didn't find anything. All your tests are normal."

I wasn't hypoglycemic. I wasn't hyperglycemic. My hormones and thyroid were fine. I didn't have Lyme disease or lupus. Blood panel? Normal. My sodium level was fine. After all that, we didn't find anything new. Except a confirmation that I had tennis elbow. From playing all that tennis, um, never. There was no reason for the pain and fatigue other than fibromyalgia.

Taryn glanced at me and then back at the floor. "It's good news, really. But I know it's not what you want to hear."

Not that I wish illness or disease upon myself, but I was

disappointed. I wanted a reason. A solution. Before I could respond, Taryn began shuffling papers into my chart.

"I could give you a prescription for pain medication?" She pulled out her prescription pad. "Or maybe you need to try counseling?"

My heart sank and tears pricked my eyes. I was losing her, the one medical professional who had been my ally. Taryn thought it was all in my head. I took a shaky breath. *How could she turn on me? How could she not believe this is real?*

"No," I said as Taryn began to slink towards the door. "I don't want any pain medication. It doesn't help and I can't afford to have too many prescriptions for pain meds in my chart." Fibromyalgia patients are sometimes stereotyped as med seeking addicts with no real pain or medical condition. "I don't want anyone to think I'm med seeking."

Taryn made eye contact, looking a little startled. "No, I know you're not med seeking. That never even crossed my mind about you."

Her hand was on the doorknob. I willed myself not to cry. "Taryn, I've done counseling. It's important to me that you believe me. I don't want to ruin the relationship I have with you, you're the best medical professional I've ever had. But I've really done counseling. This is not in my head. Counseling can't cure fibromyalgia." The tears began to drip down my face. I looked at Taryn expecting to see doubt, disgust, or even frustration.

Instead I saw tears in her eyes. She let go of the doorknob and flopped into a chair. "So, I've told you my mom has fibromyalgia, right?" She hadn't. "It's just . . . I'm sorry I can't help you. I didn't find anything we can treat. I wasn't able to help you, I can't help my mom. She's given up. She doesn't leave the house. She's addicted to pain killers. She has said her life is over." She took a breath and leaned toward me. "But you haven't given up. Don't. You keep fighting."

That was the first time I learned that chronic illness can be painful for doctors and medical professionals. It terrified me. I had always imagined being stuck at the bottom of the fibromyalgia pit by myself. Taryn was at the top with a flashlight and rope, ready to pull me out of the darkness. Now, I realized, we were in the pit together. I wanted to be back in the pit alone. I wanted to see Taryn's pinprick of light breaking into the blackness above me. I wanted her to rescue me.

But fibromyalgia isn't something I can be rescued from. I get to be my own hero by learning to live with chronic illness. But even superheroes need help. Sometimes my sidekick is a doctor or nurse practitioner. Sometimes my sidekick is a massage therapist or a chiropractor. Sometimes it's my cat. But I am in charge of the quality of my life within the boundaries of my illness. Doctors can only do so much. To help them and myself, I also need to learn how to be a good patient.

Chronically Awesome Tips:
How to be a Good Patient

- **Keep a list of any and all medications.** Note the dosage, side effects, length of time you were on the medication, and prescribing doctor.

- **Keep a list of your symptoms.** Note how often the symptoms occur, their severity, and if anything helps or hurts.

- **Keep a list of all tests and procedures.** Note the name of the procedure, the date it was performed, the requesting doctor, the doctor who does the procedure, why it was done, and the results. This includes blood tests.

- **Keep a list of any alternative treatments (including diets).** List the dates and duration, the practitioner, and your response to the treatment.

- **Bring all lists with you to any doctor's appointments.** Even if you think the office already has them.

- **Sign a release of information.** Allow your doctor to communicate with any other providers you may have.

13

BUT THIS ISN'T HOW I IMAGINED IT

Mothers are all slightly insane.
-J.D. Salinger,
The Catcher in the Rye

When Zoey was 13 months old, we were sitting in the playroom. Zoey was playing with a puzzle and drooling on some books. I was sitting in the chair with a heating pad on my neck. Zoey stood up, tickled my feet, and put my toe in her mouth. She held it firmly but gently between her teeth. I said, "NO. No biting." She looked at me, and I swear she smiled a bit. Then she bit. Hard.

My first reaction, after seeing that my toe was still attached, was anger. And not just a little bit of anger either. I went right to The Bad Place. I had visions of grabbing Zoey, shaking her, and screaming, NO BITING! I didn't do it. I left her in the playroom and walked away.

Then I sat at the table, head in my hands, and cried while Zoey screamed and raged from 15 feet away. I know that as a parent I'm not supposed to admit that I feel things like anger, let alone have visions of shaking my child.

But I did.

And I have to believe I'm not the only one.

Obviously, the line between thinking about shaking my child and actually doing it is an important one. One I have never crossed. But being in The Bad Place, being close to that

117

line, feels terrible. It is the worst of me as a person and a mother. It's one of those dirty little secrets that most people think should never be spoken. I'm tired of keeping the secret.

I know I'm supposed to say that being a mom is wonderful and that every moment with Zoey is blissful —even if I'm, like, catching her throw up in my bare hands. (True story.) I'm supposed to say that there's nothing I would rather do. In the big picture, that's true — I wouldn't trade being Zoey's mom for anything. But day-to-day? Um, it's *possible* I would rather read my book than read the picture dictionary for the 12th time. I would rather eat bonbons on the couch than change another poopy diaper. I would rather keep all my current appendages and skin intact than be bitten several times a day. Is anyone seriously going to judge me for that? Probably.

But this isn't for those people. This is for the women who tell it like it is. Motherhood is hard. We get angry. We love our children fiercely. We think bad thoughts. We show amazing restraint. We are filled up with love every time we hold our daughter's hand. We whisper to each other, "I've been there." We tell each other we're good mothers because we are. And we laugh. Sometimes a little too loud or a little too long. Maybe until we cry. We laugh because this journey is so hard and so amazing. We laugh because it's good to have company.

Pain and fatigue rob us of patience and empathy. Anger creeps closer to the surface and, sometimes, we don't think before we act. Sometimes we have to take a minute to take care of ourselves to keep our kids safe.

Chronically Awesome Tips:
What To Do When You are in The Bad Place

- **Give yourself a break.** Know that you are doing the best you can in the moment. True, this may not be your *best* moment. But that's okay. Do what you need to do to keep it from being your worst moment.

- **Take some space.** Put your kid somewhere safe (in the crib, in front of the TV, buckled in a high chair) and then take a moment to breathe or cry or lie on the floor and stare at the wall.

- **Call a friend.** Call someone who has heard you ugly cry before. Call someone who gets that some days parenting is hard as hell.

- **Call your partner.** If you are really at the end of your rope, call your partner and ask him/her to come home so you can get the space and rest you need.

- **Turn on some music.** This is an excellent time to make use of your theme song.

- **Do something to make things easier.** If that means letting your kid watch three hours of *Sesame Street*, DO IT. Remember, it is way better for your kid to watch TV than to get shaken, smacked, or screamed at.

- **Meditate.** Meditating and breathing for just three minutes will help. You may start out with clenched teeth and balled fists, but keep going. Eventually something is going to shift.

- **This too shall pass.** Remember that dealing with kids and chronic illness is like dealing with weather: Give it a minute and it will change. This awful moment will change into something else. Hopefully a better something else.

- **Do something silly.** Pour all the Cheerios in the floor and let your kid "swim" through them. Wear underwear on your head. Make up a knock-knock joke. Doing something unexpected can go a long way in lightening the mood.. So can laughter.

- **Get a change of scenery.** Go to a friend's house. Go to a drive through for milk shakes and fries. Go for a walk. Do something to change up the mood and the routine.

Being a mom and having a chronic illness is complicated. We have to balance what is best for our health with what is best for our child. Often these two things do not coincide. Again and again we have to make decisions and hope that everyone comes out whole. Except sometimes I am the one who doesn't come out whole. Or worse, sometimes my child doesn't. It's heartbreaking. We forgive and are forgiven. All of us heal. And somehow, like all parents, we just keep going.

14

FASHION POLICE

*Some days, seeing the good in all things
requires a lot more squinting than should be necessary.*
- Carly Southworth

I often see other women — in person, on Facebook, wherever
— and these other women look put together. I suspect they
have showered *and* brushed their hair. Maybe even folded and
put away their laundry before every piece of clean clothing
becomes a wrinkled mess from sitting in the laundry basket for
three days. Also, they seem to have a faint and lovely glow.
Hopefully, this glow comes from make-up and not from the
joyous, inner fulfillment of their very existence. If it's the latter,
I give up. These women, they are also wearing cute clothes.
Clothes that seem to actually *fit*. And jewelry. Beaded
necklaces, silver bracelets, dangly earrings. These put-together
women seem like they're . . . *winning*. Winning the battle against
sleep deprivation, fatigue, pain, and general momness.

I, on the other hand, am not so much winning as slogging
along. I am the epitome of frumpiness. My hair is sort of
straggly. My clothes are either too big or pull too tight in
unflattering places. It goes without saying that everything is
wrinkled. No make-up. No jewelry. I do, however, shower.
Occasionally. Sometimes I even remember to brush my hair.

Some of my disheveledness is by choice. I often don't
invest much time in my appearance (like applying make-up or
flat ironing my hair) because I would rather save my energy for

other things. I don't need to be matchy-matchy every time I go out. A hat and a ponytail often suit me just fine. I'm okay wearing fleece sweat pants to the grocery store.

The first book I ever read about living with a chronic illness suggested that we should put on make-up every day along with a set of "fresh" clothes. The theory was that we should make ourselves at least *look* good while feeling so absolutely miserable. I think this was the point where I threw the book against the wall. And injured my shoulder.

What made me so mad about the author's suggestion that I wear makeup and "fresh" clothes was that she clearly had no understanding of what it means to be fatigued. I mean *really* fatigued. On days when my energy meter is so low it could be considered nonexistent, there is no way in hell that I am going to waste valuable energy on make-up, hair, and clothes.[25] NO. WAY. I would rather play dollhouse with my daughter for 10 minutes, or read her a book while she cuddles in my lap. I would rather make myself a good breakfast. I would rather have the energy to go to my chiropractor as scheduled. I consider these things to be good investments of my energy — something that gives back to me. I will feel good having some quality time with my daughter. I will feel good if I have a healthy breakfast. I will get some pain relief from the chiropractor.

Basically, I don't care so much about looking good; I care about *feeling* good. I buy a lot of my clothes at Target, and my make-up for that matter. I can also put on my make-up in less than a minute unless I'm going somewhere fancy — lipstick and mascara take longer. Clothes are worn a couple times before washing . . . unless they smell and/or have a stain. Except for undies — those can only be worn for one day. And I loathe blow-drying my hair.

Now why, may you ask, do I not invest much time in these things? Well, because on a daily basis I find it boring and

---

[25] Having said that, I am also lucky that I am a SAHM and don't have to invest energy in these things to get ready for a paid job. You know, one where you're not going to get drooled on and peed on every day.

energy sucking. If I'm doing something special (date night with my husband, dinner at a place with tablecloths), I can bring my fancy game (or at least look appropriate), complete with flat-ironed hair. But on a regular basis? No way.

Chronically Awesome Tips:
Tricks to Looking ~~Good~~ Okayish
When You feel Bad

- **Lower your expectations.** We do not have the time, energy, or staff to look like what's-her-name on the cover of *Vogue*. Sometimes we will go to the store in sweat pants. Sometimes we will still be wearing our pajama top under our winter coat at school pick-up. Let's give ourselves a break and say that we don't have to look put together all the time.

- **Go for sporty.** Sure, one can be both sporty and stylish. But, per above, let's not set the bar too high. Sporty means we can wear yoga pants and our hair in a pony tail. Hoodies are a go! Fleece is totally acceptable! T-shirts are practically required! Sporty is my look of choice for school drop-off and pick-up.

- **Hats.** Have a cute hat for every season. Hats go a long way in hiding unwashed and/or uncombed hair.

- **Have a quick make-up routine.** When I do wear make-up, it's easy. I wear lip-gloss, powder, and blush. BAM! Done.

- **Have set outfits.** Sometimes I do have to go out even when I feel bad and have no energy. And then I turn to my Nice Outfit. Actually, I have several Nice Outfits — each at a different level of niceness. There is Casual Nice

123

(dark jeans and a semi-fitted sweater), Business Nice (pleated wool pants and a v-neck sweater), and Dressy Nice (basic black dress and flats). Not having to figure out what to wear saves me a lot of energy and stress. It's one less decision, one less thing to worry about.

- **Wear one accessory/piece of jewelry.** A cool necklace or an awesome scarf can go a long way in making me feel nice.

The point is, find out what makes you feel good. Or at least what makes you feel *better*. Is it perfume? Cute shoes? Flashy earrings? Wear it. Dress for what makes you *feel* pretty or sexy or put together. Dress for what makes you feel like you.

15

ASKING FOR HELP
FROM TOTAL STRANGERS

*If you need something from somebody,
always give that person a way to hand it to you.*
-Sue Monk Kidd,
The Secret Life of Bees

When I was diagnosed with fibromyalgia I was suddenly in the
position of having to ask anyone and everyone for help. I had
to ask for help lifting a carton of milk in the store. I had to ask
for help carrying more than a few library books. I had to ask
my husband to vacuum, lift laundry baskets, and put the frying
pan directly on the stove. I asked friends for meals and visits
and phone calls and car rides. At first, it felt horrible. Wretched
even. But I realized if I didn't ask for these things I could rarely
leave the house. Leaving the house helped me feel better. I
finally got to the point where I felt well enough to show
thanks. I dropped off cookies and chocolate covered
strawberries. I did small errands. I made casseroles. To this
day, when I am feeling well I try to do something to show
someone thanks and gratitude.

I love it when people ask me for help. I love being able to
help people back. I love being well enough to help, period. I
am finally at the point where I mostly can ask for and accept
help sort of gracefully. Sometimes friends and family like being
needed. Perhaps that's one of our chronic super powers —
helping people feel needed.

In 2008, the results of a national survey of women with

fibromyalgia were published. The study described its objective as "determin(ing) the self-reported physical function level of women with fibromyalgia."[26] Basically, they surveyed women to find out how well the women thought they themselves functioned. The conclusions? "The average woman in this sample reported having less functional ability related to activities of daily living and instrumental activities of daily living than the average community-dwelling woman in her 80s."[27]

So, let's think about this for a moment. This survey says women with like me with fibromyalgia, no matter what our age, have the physical ability of an 80 year old. Which might be cool if I was 90. But as I'm 38 I find the results of this survey to be rather . . . what's the word? Shitty.

Unfortunately, this survey feels true. I despise going to the store and being unable to lift a 12 pack of soda. I hate seeing the Crock Pot sit on our counter for four days because I have to wait for my husband to put it on the shelf. But the worst, the absolute worst, is when I can't pick up my daughter. This has happened enough that Zoey now says (on a humiliatingly regular and public basis), "My Daddy can pick me up because he is strong. But my mommy can't because she does not have the big muscles." At least whoever hears this may be left thinking I have *small* muscles which is better than no muscles, which is how it feels.

Feeling weak and fatigued and, in some cases, actually being weak, puts us in a position to (gasp!) ask for help. Here's where it gets tricky. We often don't *look* weak. We don't *look* like we have a chronic illness. We don't *look* like we need help. So we have to make stuff up. How I ask for help depends on where I am and what I need help with at the time.

There are three main places where I find I need to ask for help by making stuff up: food/retail stores, home

---

[26]Jones J, Rutledge DN, Jones KD, Matallana L, Rooks DS, "Self-assessed physical function levels of women with fibromyalgia: a national survey," *Womens Health Issues* 2008 Sep-Oct;18(5):406-12. Epub 2008 Aug 23.
[27] ibid

improvement stores, and the gym. And even though I will probably never come into contact with these people again, I just can't bring myself to tell the truth and say, "Um, I injured my shoulder peeling an orange. Can you please lift the milk into my cart?"

Chronically Awesome Tips:
How to Ask for Help From Strangers

- **Evaluate the location.** As I said, I often struggle with lifting "heavy" things, like soda or gallons of distilled water, in and out of the cart. So I scope out the aisle. Clearly, I need to go down the aisle when someone else is in the aisle or a store clerk is nearby.

- **Evaluate the ~~victim~~ helper.** If she can lift cases of soda into *her* cart, she can lift it into mine.

- **Actually ask for help.** Sorry, but you can't skip this one. "Excuse me, would you mind lifting a case of that ginger ale into my cart for me?"

- **Lie if necessary (or lie to augment your rich, imaginary inner life).** "I hurt my back moving a couch over the weekend . . ." "I totally blew out my shoulder snow boarding   . . ." "I was apprehending some dangerous criminals and got into a bit of a tussle . . ."

- **Say thank you.** I don't need to spell it out, right?

- **Give a compliment.** "You are so kind!" or "I love your coat! Red is a great color on you!"

You're done. It's a win-win. I get my soda and my unsuspecting helper-person gets to feel useful and nice/pretty/buff.

When I am ready to check-out I find that most baggers are super friendly and helpful. They are more than happy to lift the heavy stuff for me and, of course, they deserve the same thanks/compliments. If I'm at Target and need to lift something relatively major into my cart (like a rug, big mirror, etc.), I use one of those red phones to call for help. Love those phones!

I have a slightly different strategy for home improvement stores because (a) I usually need help with heavier stuff, and (b) I usually have to ask for help from men.[28] At The Home Depot I consider it a miracle if I can find what I'm looking for in the first place. So usually I have a staff person with me to show me the correct aisle and can ask him for help. However, I have to be careful with the complimenting because I don't want it to be mistaken for flirting. The goal is to get what I came for and not to be stalked by some dude from the lighting department. Telling the guy he looks good in the orange apron is out. Usually an, "Oh wow! That looked so heavy and you lifted it with one hand! Thanks!" does the trick. The other problem with these kinds of stores is that I have a heck of time lifting stuff into the trunk of my car. Which means I have to ask some random contractor guys for help in the parking lot. Sometimes they offer help when they see me struggling, which is TOTALLY AWESOME.

The gym is another place I need help. It is also often the easiest place to get help. People are there to get buff or stay buff. Usually all I have to do is make eye contact with someone with big, squeaky muscles and he/she will help me with whatever I need. Sometimes I think that these people purposely leave the 50-pound weights on the bar just so they will be asked to move it. They'll be all, "Oh geeze! Did I leave that there? I'm so sorry! Let me pick up the 50 POUNDS with my pinky finger!" Whatever. They get the job done.

Don't be afraid! Go forth and ask for help from strangers!

---

[28]Only because there seems to be a whole of a lot of them at these types of stores.

Don't come home without the four pound bag of chocolate chips from Costco because you're afraid to ask someone to lift it for you. If you're expending the energy to be out and about, you might as well get what you need.

16

GRATITUDE

*In the end, maybe it's wiser to surrender before the
miraculous scope of human generosity and to just
keep saying thank you, forever and sincerely,
for as long as we have voices.*
-Elizabeth Gilbert,
Eat, Pray, Love

It's inevitable. Dealing with chronic pain and fatigue mandates
that we lean on others. Probably more than they lean on us.
Or at least in a different way. Sometimes we lean on them so
much we drag them to the ground. Especially our families,
partners, spouses, kids, parents, siblings, and our best friends
whom we have made family. Sometimes, when we are at our
worst (our most in pain and our most fatigued), we can't be
there for them how they need us to be. This is hard for them
and us. But mostly for them.

When we are at our best and we're feeling wellish, we
need to show thanks to those people who have gotten us
through. It doesn't have to be a grand gesture (although those
are nice too), but it does have to be *something*.

I often feel like the person that fibromyalgia is hardest on
is Demetri because it affects him on a daily basis. He never
knows if he is going to be parenting solo, with a low-
functioning me, or with Mother of the Year. He never knows
when he suddenly will be responsible for all his stuff *and* all my
stuff. Even when I'm doing well he has to lift almost
everything and conform to my inability to do more than two

errands in a row. He has to let me take naps and rest so that I won't be Mean Angry Wife in the afternoon. He has to go see the early movie because I can't stay out late. He has to mow the lawn and paint all the walls of our house. He has to bring me the heating pad or the ice pack. He has to make me hot tea. He has to put Zoey to bed *again* because I am too tired. He has to lift our 40-pound daughter in and out of everything because my back hurts. He has to give me time to exercise so my pain level stays low. He has to skip a family get-together because I'm fatigued and not up for large groups. He has to travel less. He has to drive whenever we're in the car together. He has to alter his life in a billion other ways that I'm not even aware of.

I try to remember all of this. I try to thank him every single day for what he does. But sometimes I don't. Often I take him for granted. Because he is kind, he never points this out to me. But I know it has to hurt. So, LET THE RECORD SHOW: MY HUSBAND ROCKS AND I ADORE HIM. EVERY. SINGLE. DAY.

Chronically Awesome Lists:
Ways To Show Thanks, Appreciation, and Gratitude

- **Send a card** (funny, sappy, handmade, whatever).
- **Cook a meal** for your partner or drop off take-out for a friend. People love not having to cook — especially people with small, whiny children.
- **Drop off a treat.** Chocolate covered strawberries, chocolate croissants, a bar of chocolate.
- **Make an appreciation list** of all the reasons you appreciate your friend/partner and then show it to him.
- **Send flowers.**
- **Pass on a book or magazine** you know your friend will like.

132

- **Ask how you can help** and then help (or get the help your friend/partner needs).
- **Take him to lunch/breakfast.**
- **Make a mix CD.**
- **Hug everyone.**
- **Say, "Thank you."** Look your partner/freind in the eyes and mean it.
- **Be kind** (don't let your pain and fatigue do the talking).
- **Perform an interpretive dance** (scarves are optional).
- **Give your partner time and permission to do something for him/herself.**
- **Tell your friend/partner what you wish you could do for them.** If you can't do any of these things because your energy/pain just won't allow it, do an I Wish List: "I wish I could send you to Hawaii for two weeks and have fresh pineapple delivered to you on the beach every day by a hot cabana boy in too-tight shorts."
- **Do something.** Say something. Try not to let things go without saying thanks.

CONCLUSION

Life is not so much about beginnings and endings
as it is about going on and on and on.
It is about muddling through the middle.
- Anna Quindlen

As I'm writing this, I'm coming off a stressful week that was full of fibromyalgia pain and fatigue. I am so very aware of the truly delicate balance that it takes to feel well. Most of all I am reminded that I need to be gentle with myself; I need to work with where I am now, not where I wish I was. And often this week I wished my body was in a different place — a stronger place.

Right now I am building up, lying low, and reaching for a bit more energy every day. I am exercising and meditating and seeing the chiropractor. I am doing my physical therapy exercises and saying "no" to things I really would like to do. I am refusing to lift anything over five pounds. I am cooking easy meals and not cleaning the house. I am resting. I am letting myself feel a little sad and a little small. And I am letting myself know, *This too shall pass.*

My wish is that this book made you smile and gave you hope. Maybe you even feel less alone. Chronic illness is not something we have to go through in isolation.

Tell everyone about fibromyalgia, lupus, IBS, MS, depression — whatever your chronic illness is. Then tell them that you are still you. You are still funny and wacky and smart and a total hottie. You are a super hero. Don't ever forget it.

OTHER RESOURCES

How To Be Sick: A Buddhist-Inspired Guide for the Chronically Ill and Their Caregivers by Toni Bernhard

The Chronically Awesome Foundation
http://chronicallyawesome.org/

Invisible Disabilities Association
http://invisibledisabilities.org/

Mayo Clinic: Diseases and Conditions
Comprehensive guides on hundreds of conditions
http://www.mayoclinic.org/diseases-conditions

National Fibromyalgia Association
http://www.fmaware.org/

National Fibromyalgia & Chronic Pain Association
http://www.fmcpaware.org/

WORKS CITED

"About Chronic Diseases." *nationalhealthcouncil.org.* Last modified April 11, 3013. http://www.nationalhealthcouncil. org/ NHC_Files/Pdf_Files/AboutChronicDisease.pdf.

Bennett, Robert. "Newly Diagnosed Patient." FMaware.org, accessed February 14, 2014. http://www.fmaware.org/ PageServer0bbc.html? pagename=fibromyalgia_overview.

Deffner, Elisabeth, "Get a Better Night's Sleep," *Fibromyalgia Aware*, Spring 2009: 14.

Dupree Jones, Kim and Janice Holt Hoffman, "Exercise and Chronic Pain: Opening the Therapeutic Window, *Functional*, Volume 1, Number 4, January-February 2006. http://www. myalgia.com/Exercise/ICAA_Functionalu_Vol4_1.pdf.

"Fibromyalgia (FMS)." *Arthritis.org.* Accessed February 13, 2014. http://www.arthritis.org/conditions-treatments/disease-center/fibromyalgia-fms/.

Jones J, Rutledge DN, Jones KD, Matallana L, Rooks DS, "Self-assessed physical function levels of women with fibromyalgia: a national survey," *Womens Health Issues 2008 Sep-Oct;18(5):406-12. Epub 2008 Aug 23.*

Kubler-Ross, Elisabeth. "On Death and Dying." (New York: Scribner, 1969).

Longley, Kathy. "My Kingdom for a Good Night's Sleep," reprinted from *FMOnline*, June 21, 2007, www.fmaware.org/ News2ffa1.html?page= NewsArticle&id=5367.

Matallana, Lynne. "Depression and Fibromyalgia," reprinted from FMOnline, October 1, 2006. http://www.fmaware.org/ News289e4.html?page= NewsArticle&id=6229.

Mayo Clinic Staff. "Definition." *Diseases and Conditions: Fibromyalgia.* Accessed January 22, 2011. http://www.mayo clinic.org/diseases-conditions/fibromyalgia/basics/definition /CON-20019243.

Melkerson, MN. "Special Premarket 510(k) Notification for NeuroStar TMS Therapy System for Major Depressive Disorder" (pdf). Food and Drug Administration. December 16, 2008. http://www.accessdata.fda.gov/cdrh_docs /pdf8/K083538.pdf.

"Mindfulness Meditation: A New Treatment For Fibromyalgia?." *Sciencedaily.com*, accessed February 13, 2014. http://www.sciencedaily.com/releases/2007/08/ 070805134742.htm.

"Pilates." *Wikipedia.org.* http://en.wikipedia.org/wiki/Pilates.

"Symptoms." Depression (Maror Depressive Disorder). *Mayoclinic.org.* Retrieved August 10, 2013. http://www. mayoclinic.org/diseases-conditions/ depression/ basics/symptoms/con-20032977.

"The Faces of Fibromyalgia." May 2011, *fibrocenter.com*, retrieved August 2, 2012, http://www.fibrocenter.com/media/ Faces_of_Fibromyalgia_Factsheet.pdf .

"The Five Stages of Grief The responses to Grief that Many People Have." *Grief.com.* Retrieved June 28, 2013. http://grief. com/the-five-stages-of-grief/.

Joslyne is a mother of one and is currently a fighter of fibromyalgia, depression, and some weird bilateral foot pain that has the doctors stumped. She spends part of every day looking for chocolate her husband hides for her. He either has a lot of really good hiding places or Joslyne forgets where—wait, what was she looking for again? Joslyne lives outside of Boston with Demetri, Zoey, and various pets. Check out her blog at joslynedecker.wordpress.com.

Made in the USA
Monee, IL
10 February 2020

21568373R00085